THE PREGNANCY HANDBOOK FOR FIRST-TIME MOMS

A COMPREHENSIVE GUIDE COVERING WEEKLY FETAL DEVELOPMENT, MATERNAL CHANGES, PRENATAL TESTS, AND MAKING INFORMED DECISIONS

LINDA TOURVILLE MSN

PARENTHOOD PRESS

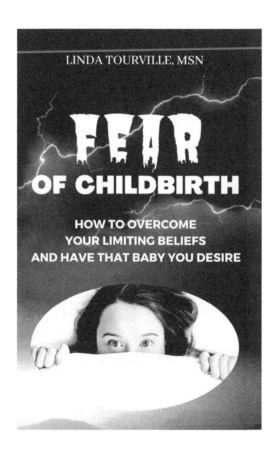

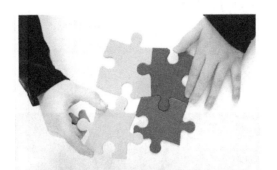

PARENTING
YOUR CHILD WITH
AUTISM

PRACTICAL STRATEGIES TO MEET THE CHALLENGES
AND HELP YOUR FAMILY THRIVE

LUCY TALBOTT

CONTENTS

Introduction   xi

PART I

1. A NEW BEGINNING   3
   The Importance of Women-Centered Care   4
   Pregnancy Is A Sacred Experience   7
   Be Prepared for Big Changes   12
   Chapter Summary   13

2. RIGHTS, OPTIONS, AND DECISIONS   15
   Pregnant Patient's Bill of Rights   15
   Making Informed Decisions   19
   Types of Birth   20
   Choosing the Place of Birth   24
   Choosing a Healthcare Provider   26
   Chapter Summary   27

PART II

3. TAKING CARE OF YOUR HEALTH DURING
   PREGNANCY   31
   Foods to Enjoy and Foods to Avoid During Your
   Pregnancy   31
   Staying Active During Your Pregnancy   33
   Maintaining Your Back Health   35
   Sex During Pregnancy   36
   Getting a Good Night's Sleep   37
   Maintaining Good Dental Health   39
   Avoiding Harmful Substances   40
   Working During Your Pregnancy   41
   Will Your Pregnancy Affect Your Travel Plans?   42
   Pregnancy and Pets   42
   Chapter Summary   43

4. COMMON CONCERNS AND DISCOMFORTS   45
Breast Tenderness and Other Changes   45
Constipation   46
Dreams   47
Fatigue During Pregnancy   47
Frequent Urination   48
Headaches   49
Heartburn   51
Hemorrhoids   51
Increased Vaginal Discharge   52
Itchy Skin   53
Leg Cramps   54
Mood Changes   55
Morning Sickness   55
Round Ligament Pain   56
Shortness of Breath   57
Swollen Fingers, Ankles, and Feet   58
Uterine Cramping   59
Varicose Veins   60
Chapter Summary   61

PART III

5. THE FIRST TRIMESTER   65
Fetal Growth and Development During the First
Trimester   66
Maternal Body Changes During the First Trimester   77
Emotional Changes During the First Trimester   79
Your First Prenatal Visit   82
Chapter Summary   85

6. THE SECOND TRIMESTER   87
Fetal Growth and Development During the Second
Trimester   88
Maternal Body Changes During the Second Trimester   100
Emotional Changes During the Second Trimester   102
Your Week 16 Prenatal Visit   103
Your Week 20 Prenatal Visit   104
Your Week 24 Prenatal Visit   105
Chapter Summary   106

7. THE THIRD TRIMESTER   107
   Fetal Growth and Development During the Third
   Trimester   108
   Maternal Body Changes During the Third Trimester   123
   Emotional Changes During the Third Trimester   124
   Your Week 28 Prenatal Visit   124
   Your Prenatal Visits in Weeks 30, 32, and 34   125
   Your Week 36 Prenatal Visit   126
   Your Prenatal Visits in Weeks 37, 38, 39, and 40   126
   Your Week 41 Prenatal Visit   127
   Chapter Summary   127

   Conclusion   129
   Also Available From Parenthood Press   133
   References   135

For my exceptional daughters,
without whom
I wouldn't have found
a deeper meaning to birthin' babies.

Marm

INTRODUCTION

You may forget many important events, such as the day you met your best friend or your first day at work. Still, one memory that will probably remain crystal clear throughout your lifetime is the moment you found out you were pregnant. This life-changing news is always impactful. You can hear many funny, emotional, and sad stories about the moment women realized they were pregnant. Some women waited for years to experience pregnancy and wept for joy when they discovered the news. While others, stunned by how quickly they got pregnant, suddenly felt a bout of "morning sickness" even though they took their pregnancy test just that afternoon or evening. And others, knowing that a pregnancy at this time in their lives was a problem, did not welcome the news.

When you first tell others you are pregnant, be prepared for a barrage of advice. There is perhaps no other time in your life in which others will be more interested in helping you, sharing their knowledge with you, or, in some cases, advising you on the best course of action. Don't be taken aback if you are a few weeks pregnant and people are already giving you advice on everything from epidurals to episiotomies.

Meet Breonna, who feels a little overwhelmed by information over-load. She never really let others steer her away from her chosen path. She listened to what her partner, friends, and loved ones had to say. Breonna ultimately made a detailed pregnancy plan based on the evidence she obtained from her reading, the advice of her midwife, and the information she had received in prenatal classes. She enjoyed speaking with her best friend, mainly because they shared views on natural birth, pregnancy massage, and the importance of nurturing oneself during pregnancy.

Breonna never let insecurity or a lack of knowledge about pregnancy stand in her way. She armed herself with information, spoke with many people, researched the interesting points others brought up, and listened to her instincts. While there are studies on everything from what medications are safe during pregnancy to cleaning the cat litter box, you must choose what is right for yourself. This can only be done when you know your mind and body and make your choices coura-geously, without fear.

This book intends to empower you to make your own choices after knowing all your rights and options. One of the biggest mistakes you can make is entering the birthing experience believing your body is a passive vessel and saying "yes" to everything proposed to you. Saying "no" is always a choice. You should know you have a wide range of options before, during, and after delivery.

Of course, entrusting your birth to a team you trust is critical to developing the confidence you need to make the right decisions for you and your baby. While an obstetrician will always recommend courses of action that protect you and your baby, many choices you can make will impact the birthing process and your ability to recover and bond with your baby.

Choosing a team that respects your views and beliefs and has the required medical expertise is one of the most critical steps. Commu-nicating well with your team is necessary. Preparing a detailed birth plan ensures they are familiar with your preferences, concerns, values, life experiences, and beliefs in the months leading up to your baby's birth.

Carefully consider the options presented to you and make your decisions based on evidence, not beliefs and stories. There is immense value in seeing pregnancy as an extraordinary moment in your life. Pregnancy is not something to grind through, nor is it a competition with yourself or others. While it can sometimes be reduced to an almost clinical experience that is necessary to bring new life into the world, it can also be a spiritual experience that profoundly affects mothers, fathers, partners, and entire families.

This book will share tips, the experiences of mothers, and an idea of what pregnancy can be if you make the most of it. There will arguably never be another time when your body, mind, and spirituality will feel so united and be so determinative of your decisions. Therefore, it is important to invest time and effort in good prenatal care. In prenatal classes, relax and experience calming sensations while connecting with other mothers.

When choosing a group to share your life, fears, joys, thoughts, and beliefs with, make sure it affirms who you are. Acceptance, openness, and respect for differences should coexist. Prenatal classes should not simply delve into scientific matters such as pregnancy tests, diets, and legal rights. They should encourage you to talk about how you feel, empower you to feel more closely connected to life and nature, and celebrate this special time of grace.

Daily life is busy and fraught with expectations, demands, and responsibilities. Some women work non-stop until practically the day of their baby's birth. They did not take the time they needed to understand and respect the seismic shift that carrying a life in one's womb can be.

This book will delve into pregnancy's practicalities, including the rights, options, and decisions to be considered. You will have many decisions to make, so take it slow and give yourself time to read, talk to others, and strengthen your inner resolve. These can range from the type of birth you choose to where you will be giving birth—at home, in a hospital, or at a birth center. There is no ideal path that suits everyone equally.

Take a healthy approach to pregnancy by exercising self-kindness, eating healthily, and following practical tips, such as how to prevent back pain and the importance of good dental health during pregnancy. You will read about common concerns and discomforts and get advice on how to overcome them, if possible. For instance, one frequent complaint is heartburn, which you can easily remedy by avoiding certain foods.

After many months of discussing an array of pregnancy-related subjects with loved ones, the final trimester of your pregnancy is an excellent time to make critical decisions. These include preparing to breastfeed or use a bottle; deciding on options for labor pain management; writing a birth plan; purchasing baby equipment; and planning your postpartum support network.

The last three chapters of this book will immerse you in what to expect during the three trimesters of pregnancy. Subjects such as fetal development, bodily and emotional changes, routine prenatal care, and important tests will be covered.

You will feel more knowledgeable, decisive, and confident when you finish reading this book. Take a proactive approach to your pregnancy. Read material that empowers you, surround yourself with supportive people, and savor every moment of this deeply sacred and uniquely beautiful experience.

PART I

If you don't know your options, you don't have any.

— DIANA KORTE

Pregnancy is a time of significant change. You are growing a new life, and you must ensure you are prepared for all the changes you will be experiencing. This can be difficult when you don't know your options, so it is essential to make sure you do your research to make informed decisions. When you know all of your options, it will be much easier to decide which one is best for you.

As you weigh your options, keep in mind that there is no one right way to have a baby. It may be essential for you to make peace with your personal preferences about what is best for you and your family.

Take responsibility for making decisions about your care. Don't hesitate to ask questions and seek out information from trusted sources when in doubt. There's no reason you have to feel like you're lost in the shuffle when taking charge of your health care.

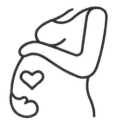

1

A NEW BEGINNING

From the time you were a child, you've probably heard many women share their experiences of pregnancy, with some referring to the birth of their child as life-changing. Most new moms become flooded with emotions, and tears of joy are nearly always involved. This is a moment you will never forget, and it will powerfully change your life.

Becoming a mother is a challenge for your body. It is an awakening. For example, right after you give birth, estrogen and progesterone levels drop dramatically, leading to baby blues, sadness, or even post-partum depression (Schiedel, 2018). This is why you should empower yourself, take care of yourself, and make choices that make you feel safe during pregnancy.

The more you feel you have had a say in your pregnancy and delivery, the less likely you feel like you are a passive vessel for others' decisions. Advice from experienced, trained medical professionals is always essential, and evidence should be the overriding factor when making key decisions. However, respecting your individual beliefs, thoughts, and values is important. The professionals you rely on should be interested in learning more about you and accommodating your needs and wishes as much as possible.

THE IMPORTANCE OF WOMEN-CENTERED CARE

You have the right to seek prenatal, birth, and postpartum care that is medically safe and recognizes your individual psychological, cultural, spiritual, physical, and economic needs. Woman-centered care focuses on your unique needs, wishes, and expectations. It recognizes your right to self-determination in choice, control, and continued care. It additionally acknowledges that you and your baby, whether born or unborn, are part of their social and emotional environment. Understanding and respecting your individuality should be a key pillar in providing you with care (Australian Government Department of Health, n.d.).

Taking Cultural Safety Into Account

Cultural safety is an approach that seeks to incorporate cultural awareness and sensitivity into health care. Different cultures can view pregnancy and birth very differently. For example, birth is accepted as a natural process in countries like New Zealand. The mother is physically prepared to care for her baby from birth with minimal intervention and assistance.

In contrast, many cultures view maternity as a vulnerable period that requires frequent surveillance, monitoring, rest, and nurturing before the mother can take on new duties (De Souza, 2016). In these cultures, the new mother becomes a caregiver by receiving care herself. Thus, postpartum practices can include receiving organized support from friends and loved ones, resting from work and sex for a specific time, consuming a special diet with healing foods, and the like. Beliefs and practices can vary greatly depending on your social context.

Your social context impacts subjects such as infant care and breastfeeding, maternal massage, and belly binding, which involves wrapping a belly to provide physical and emotional support. Belly binding supports the back (At First Sight, n.d.) and boosts good posture. Some women describe it as "a big hug" that is highly soothing (NLBS Admin Team, 2020).

Many cultures across the globe have postpartum confinement periods. In the Mexican tradition of "cuarentena," the new mom abstains from sex and dedicates herself exclusively to breastfeeding and caring for her baby and herself for 40 days. During this period, family members take care of tasks like cooking, tidying up the home, and caring for any other children in the household. Women avoid drafts of air because, during this period, the body is considered "open" and vulnerable. The traditions of the cuarentena help "close" the body (Waugh, 2011), which is the main aim of postpartum recovery. Health providers need to recognize your specific beliefs and customs since failing to do so can be a barrier to you seeking appropriate health care.

You Have the Right and Duty to Take an Active Role in Your Healthcare

According to research by the National Council on Patient Information and Education, around 92% of US citizens prefer having better health control (Klick Wire Editor, 2015). Meanwhile, national surveys undertaken in the UK show 40% of people would like to be more involved in decisions about their care (NHS England, n.d.). During pregnancy, women wish to take responsibility for their well-being. Those with midwives have stated they want to have professional support from their midwives when they transition into motherhood (Seefat-van Teefelen et al., 2009).

There are many strategies you can use to be proactive during pregnancy. You may prioritize different aspects. You may want to write out a pregnancy plan when you are in your first trimester. You may focus on eating healthier and exercising. In reality, all these approaches should coexist since pregnancy encompasses various areas of your health. The choices you make can impact your baby's health.

Being proactive extends to actively avoiding exposure to dangerous toxins, chemicals, and foods that can harm your baby. These include high-mercury fish, raw fish, undercooked meats, and raw hams, which risk toxoplasmosis. This infection can cause premature birth and other health problems.

Pregnancy is an excellent time to learn, educate yourself, talk to health professionals, and be brave enough to ask the questions that may be troubling you. It is a time when sticking to recommended health provider visits, including postpartum visits, is vital. For example, Carmen was reluctant to keep these appointments. She was very focused on her baby and thought attending postpartum visits was a waste of her time. She experienced no complications during the birth, and her baby was thriving. A few months later, Carmen was worried she had postpartum depression.

Postpartum doula care can be an option for you. An experienced doula helps with so many aspects that can interfere with your postpartum experience. They can provide breastfeeding support, help with the care of your newborn, and aid in your emotional and physical recovery. Attending postpartum visits with your medical team is vital because seasoned professionals are trained to look for signs of issues that need addressing. Additionally, they can answer questions about breastfeeding, recommend vitamin supplementation, and more.

Childbirth Is a Normal, Healthy Experience

Caregivers must support and promote the health of you and your baby. They must be confident about the normality of childbirth and be ready to recognize and address deviations from the norm that could potentially harm you or your baby.

Information Is Vital and Should Be Shared

Patients, doctors, midwives, and other members of the birthing team should actively seek information and freely share their findings. Share this information with your family, since family members can provide crucial support in the prenatal, pregnancy, and postpartum stages.

You Define Who to Include as Family

You should decide who your "family" members are for your pregnancy and delivery. You alone should determine who you want to be present during the moment of birth and who to rely on in the months leading up to this crucial period. These family members should take on shared responsibility and make choices alongside you when appropriate.

PREGNANCY IS A SACRED EXPERIENCE

Pregnancy can be one of the most transformative moments in your life since it involves seismic shifts in your physical, mental, and emotional states. Too often, pregnancy is focused exclusively on the physical—making appointments on time, completing each testing stage, and dealing with the changes that pregnancy physically produces. However, opening yourself up to the spiritual nature of pregnancy can help make it a more meaningful and richer experience.

Those who see the sacrament of birth as sacred understand that they are bringing a new soul into the plane of existence. Some women who may not have been deeply religious or valued spirituality in their daily lives made a significant transformation during their pregnancy. This change helped them slow down, take stock of their emotions, and understand that their relationship with their partner was also changing.

In the past, women gathered with their sisters to honor their baby's first breaths of life. Today, this sense of group support may be missing. Women may need to search for it in other places—including yoga groups, prenatal classes, and sacred massage.

You don't have to believe in a specific religion to be spiritual. Spirituality consists of being aware you are part of something larger than yourself—it could be a life force or energy that grounds you in love and compassion (Motherhood Community, 2021). While some moms choose to see their body as mainly a physical vessel that nurtures and protects the baby growing within them, others see pregnancy as their transformation into a protector, creator, and keeper. Pregnancy becomes the ultimate symbol of your unity with the powerful life force that unites all sentient beings.

Embracing Holistic Practices

Tapping into the sacred side of your pregnancy through holistic practices like Kundalini yoga, meditation, or exercise can make you feel calm and confident about everything from the birthing experience to how you connect with your partner and/or other friends and family members. These techniques, meditations, and exercises have been handed down from generation to generation. They amount to the spiritual wisdom women have taught each other for centuries.

Healing Past Hurts

Pregnancy can be an ideal time to heal wounds and end the burden that past trauma, such as feeling unloved as a child, has had on our lives. As a future mother, you can make different choices than those made for you. You can choose to do the inner work you require to know yourself better and identify your strengths and limitations.

Your heightened self-awareness can help motivate you to read up on aspects such as emotional regulation, anger management, how to de-stress, and other strategies that can help you make more elevated choices and give your baby the gift of your calm, healing, and wholeness. It can strengthen you and make you feel like a warrior who is neither bound by the past nor worried about what could happen in the future.

You are a powerful protector of your child and yourself. You can weather any storm that arises while knowing the importance of support and professional help when needed.

Harnessing the Power of Sacred Touch

Pregnancy massage is a way for you to remember your sacredness, your role as a creator, and your ability to connect in a powerful way to the Earth. Suzanne Yates (2017), a sacred pregnancy advocate, recalls a Buddhist monk who once told her the most important moments in our lives can be considered "deep drinks from the well of life," and pregnancy is the deepest of these sips. It is considered "a nine-month meditation." Experience pregnancy in a quiet, calm way through holistic practices. These can be as simple as controlled breathing in a beautiful natural spot, taking part in an outdoor pregnancy yoga class, or taking a "forest bath," opening your senses to the majesty and vastness of nature.

Sacred pregnancy massage is a powerful way to honor, nurture, and encourage yourself to feel the power of this moment in your life; it can transform you and make you feel more powerful, while also making you infinitely kinder.

Massage during pregnancy is beneficial for both you and your growing fetus. Gentle pressure on the abdomen encourages blood flow to the baby, providing essential nutrients and oxygen. Additionally, the growing bump is incredibly sensitive and prone to stretch marks. Massaging it during pregnancy can reduce these appearances over time.

Many cultures incorporate touch into the rituals that surround pregnancy. For instance, some Jamaican midwives rub a mother's body with olive oil or unique leaves or use a warm cloth to pat the belly to ease the pain. Meanwhile, throughout Central America, Mayan therapeutic uterine massage is used to relax the solar plexus and realign the uterus into the desired anatomical position. It is done on the upper abdomen, above the top of the uterus, to balance overstretched muscles and ligaments and alleviate symptoms of indigestion (Descisciolo, 2017).

Touch can bring you great comfort. A gentle backrub, embrace, or massage can help you feel nurtured, accompanied, and supported. Touch and massage are powerful ways to pass on the wisdom of generations through symbolic gestures. Receiving a sacred massage reminds you of the importance of nurturing your child through touch. Research indicates newborns who receive nurturing touch grow faster and show improved motor skills and mental development (The Spring, 2022). Children who receive affection are less aggressive.

Couples who cuddle have lower stress levels, better immunity, and lower blood pressure than those who do not receive nurturing touch or physical affection.

Choosing a Midwife With a Spiritual Understanding

If you wish to make spirituality an essential part of your pregnancy and motherhood, consider working with a midwife who values aspects such as stillness, breathing, holistic relaxation, and connecting with your baby through visualization that can help you achieve your goal. Your midwife should have a deep love for and commitment to women and make you feel like a sister, not just a patient. When they see your body as a sacred vessel, they can help encourage you to maintain a loving attitude towards your body, mind, and spirit while pregnant. It is vital to feel positive, empowered, and beautiful about the changes in your body—to embrace the graceful curves that symbolize your role as nurturer and protector.

Your midwife should notice signs of worry and distress, which can manifest themselves, for example, through your breathing pattern. She can teach you to release these fears or concerns through breathing techniques or sound. Sometimes, all you need to feel better on a day you feel low is someone who sees and hears you, giving you 100% of themselves and venturing to enter into your "here and now." When you feel genuinely cared for by someone like your midwife, you feel more open to talking about your concerns and releasing tension through tears and even laughter.

Your family can play an essential role in your spiritual journey. If you have a partner or spouse, they may wish to attend a sacred massage session and learn a few techniques they can impart or take part in alongside you at home. Your midwife can teach your partner or another loved one, for instance, how to use touch to soothe you during labor, such as massaging your back.

By including your partner or other loved ones in your transformation, you can feel reaffirmed in your new role as a vessel of life and the carrier of a new soul. You can learn how to give healing massages to your loved ones. The power of touch goes both ways; it always unites and boosts feelings of love, empathy, and kindness.

Here are some examples of how a few women chose to prepare themselves more fully for a sacred pregnancy:

I embraced various holistic practices from my first trimester onward. I battled (and still do) against anxiety, so I needed to choose powerful, tried-and-tested healing methods. I opted for Kundalini yoga and made it a point to walk to the park and enjoy time sitting outdoors and practicing controlled breathing exercises. To feel more nurtured, I chose Reiki. I found that it calmed and relaxed me and helped me let go of fears, anxieties, and negative feelings.

— GRETA, A BUSINESS OWNER AND MOTHER OF
THREE

∼

I read many books and spoke to many people, but I decided very early on not to compare myself to other moms and not to feel guilty if I did not do everything I was advised to do.

— ELLA, A JOURNALIST AND MOTHER OF ONE

∼

I decided to trust my instincts. There were many things I thought I should be doing, like yoga, but I found that I experienced backaches and went with my instinct. After giving birth, I tried yoga again and have become an active practitioner. For some reason, pregnancy was not the right time for yoga, though many of my friends loved it and reaped big

rewards. For me, it's all about listening to yourself and going with what
feels right for you.

— LAURA, A FREELANCE WRITER AND MOTHER
OF ONE

___

BE PREPARED FOR BIG CHANGES

The many physical changes you are about to experience can change
how you think, feel, or behave. Understand these changes and share
them with your loved ones (Kids Health, n.d.). Just a few of the
changes pregnancy can bring include:

- **Hormonal Changes**: These can result in problems with
  concentration and can cause mood swings.
- **Honing the Nesting Instinct**: Many pregnant women feel a
  strong urge to get their homes ready for their babies. They
  may develop a stronger interest in home decor, baby furniture
  and accessories, and may prioritize tidiness more.
- **Physical Changes**: Breast growth occurs quickly in the first
  trimester due to a surge in estrogen and progesterone levels,
  though your breasts can continue to grow throughout the
  pregnancy. You can experience various skin changes. Blood
  volume increases during pregnancy, bringing more blood to
  the vessels and increasing oil gland secretion. This can lead to
  what is known as "pregnancy acne."

You may notice additional changes, such as the development of a
brown line, the linea nigra, that runs down from below the chest to
the bottom of the abdomen. Or the line can start more or less at the
belly button and reach the pubis. You may develop brown or
yellowish patches on your face known as melasma, also known as "the
mask of pregnancy." You can develop a heat rash or experience itchiness as the skin starts to stretch. You can experience substantial hair

growth and stronger nails. These changes are due to hormonal fluctuations and are temporary.

When you are pregnant, you may develop swollen feet and varicose veins. Hemorrhoids and constipation may become bothersome. All these issues have specific causes. For instance, hemorrhoids can occur because blood volume increases. The uterus can exert more pressure on the pelvis, causing the rectal veins to form clusters. Constipation, meanwhile, can occur for hormonal reasons. It can also happen because, in the later stages of pregnancy, the uterus can push against the intestine, making it harder to have bowel movements. To prevent hemorrhoids and constipation, aim to consume a Mediterranean fiber-rich diet, drink plenty of water, and exercise daily.

CHAPTER SUMMARY

Pregnancy is a special time in life. Make it a meaningful, empowering experience by:

- embracing a woman-centered approach to your pregnancy
- relying on a team that takes your cultural safety into account
- taking an active role in the care you receive
- seeing childbirth as a normal, healthy experience
- encouraging your family to form a support network
- taking a sacred approach to pregnancy and embracing holistic practices
- seeing pregnancy as motivation to heal old wounds
- choosing a healthcare provider who prioritizes the spiritual significance of pregnancy
- knowing what to expect and share information about key changes with those you love

Chapter Two will highlight specific topics such as the pregnant patient's bill of rights, making informed decisions about the different options you have, choosing your health care provider and a place for your delivery, and other key subjects.

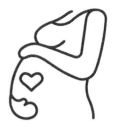

RIGHTS, OPTIONS, AND DECISIONS

Access to a wide range of information is vital if you want to make the best choices for your baby's birth and beyond. This chapter will take you through your rights and options, covering topics such as informed consent, the type and place of birth, and your chosen provider.

PREGNANT PATIENT'S BILL OF RIGHTS

The concern for pregnant women's rights began in the 1950s when the natural childbirth movement began to gain ground. Problems arose regarding some practices employed during childbirth. These practices included performing procedures and administering medications that were not always necessary and could potentially harm a mother and her baby. Consumer and health-related groups began to advocate for a pregnant woman's right to give informed consent for procedures relating to childbirth.

These groups were concerned because there was a lack of information regarding how specific treatments and medications could cause oxygen depletion, changes in brain chemistry, fractures due to forceps, and more. They noted that a drug's being approved by the FDA does not necessarily mean it is safe for an unborn child.

In 1974, the American College of Obstetricians and Gynecologists (ACOG) recognized that physicians had a legal obligation to obtain informed consent before treatment. It did so via the publication of the Standards for Obstetric-Gynecologic Services (Alliance for the Improvement of Maternity Services, n.d.).

Learning the Difference Between Consent and Informed Consent

The Standards for Obstetric-Gynecologic Services stipulate "consent" and "informed consent" are different. Many doctors thought they would be free of liability if they had a patient's consent. The new standards made it clear that the physician had a duty to obtain informed consent. That is, they had to give the following information to their patients:

- the processes involved in treatment, including when therapies are novel or unusual
- the reasons why a specific treatment is offered
- the risks and benefits involved
- the chances for recovery post-treatment
- how necessary the treatment was
- the feasibility of other types of treatment

It mattered how healthcare providers gave explanations. Physicians needed to act with due care, ensuring the patient understood what was being explained. The new standards are deemed insufficient to justify failing to provide expected information for specific reasons. Some of these reasons included (a) a patient not wanting to know unpleasant possibilities regarding the treatment and (b) a physician thinking their patient would refuse treatment if they were aware of the risks involved.

What Rights Can You Expect as a Pregnant Patient?

The standards delineate various rights. In essence, as a pregnant patient, you have the right to expect:

- information about the potential direct and indirect risks to yourself as a mother or to your unborn child because of specific procedures and medications
- an explanation of the benefits, risks, and alternatives to a treatment being suggested or discussed
- information about the effects a medication may have on your unborn child—this includes the disclosure of uncertainties regarding how a drug may affect your child's physical, mental, or neurological development
- in the case of cesarean delivery, instruction that minimal use of non-essential preoperative drugs is beneficial
- information about the brand and generic names of all drugs
- the right to select a preferred procedure and its inherent risks without pressure
- information about whether a medication or procedure is beneficial or merely elective
- the right to choose your position during labor while receiving appropriate medical advice
- the right to have your baby cared for by your bedside unless complications are present
- the right to be accompanied during labor and delivery by someone you care for
- written identification of the physician who delivers your baby
- disclosure of any care-related aspect that could lead to subsequent difficulties
- the right to have the hospital keep accurate, legible records until your newborn reaches maturity or to have these records sent to you before they are eliminated
- the right to access records by paying a reasonable fee, without legal aid

If any of these rights are not respected and injury arises, there could be grounds for a medical malpractice case (Legal Match, n.d.).

What Rights Do You Have to Refuse Treatment?

One of the biggest challenges for physicians is when a patient refuses to receive medical treatment that aims to support her and her baby's well-being. Your physician has the ethical obligation to safeguard your autonomy, which may conflict with the ethical wish to protect you and your baby's health. The American College of Obstetricians and Gynecologists (ACOG, 2019) recommends the following:

- A pregnant patient has the same right to refuse recommended medications or surgical procedures as all other patients. The physician should respect this right—even if the treatment or procedure is necessary to maintain life.
- Obstetrician-gynecologists (OB-GYNs) should never use coercion, threats, manipulation, or physical force to influence a pregnant patient toward a clinical decision.
- An OB-GYN cannot use "conscience" to justify attempting to coerce a patient into receiving treatment she does not want.
- When working to reach a resolution with a pregnant patient who has refused a recommended treatment, consideration should be given to factors such as the seriousness of the possible outcome, the extent to which the patient understands the potential severity of the risk involved, and the degree of urgency. Ultimately, the patient should be reassured that her wishes will be respected if she refuses treatment recommendations.
- ACOG opposes the use of courts to force medical interventions on unwilling patients.
- ACOG discourages medical institutions from seeking court-ordered interventions or punishing OBG-GYNs who refuse to perform them.
- OB-GYNs should aim to resolve conflicts via a team approach, seeking advice from ethics consultants when they, or the patient, feel this will help.
- Resources should be provided to patients with adverse outcomes after refusing recommended treatment.

Even in cases in which physicians are deeply concerned about the health of you and your fetus, their actions should be guided by the ethical principle that adult patients capable of making decisions have the right to refuse medical treatment.

MAKING INFORMED DECISIONS

Because your decisions can significantly impact your well-being and that of your baby, you must make informed decisions. This means you should proactively seek information on all aspects of your pregnancy and use it to make critical choices during your pregnancy (Childbirth Connection, n.d.). Research risks and benefits, ask and answer questions, and share your preferences with your health care providers and support network. While you will find conflicting information and an oversupply of advice, it is vital to base your decisions on scientific evidence, studies, and other types of recently published research.

Choosing Evidence-Based Maternity Care

Not all evidence has the same quality. A large-scale study involving thousands of cases, for instance, has more "weight" than a small-scale study or an anecdotal report. To make evidence-based decisions, weigh the merits of the studies you read, question common assumptions, and give due weight to high-quality research.

Talking With Your Maternity Care Provider

Bring all the information you have obtained to your discussions with your maternity care provider. List any questions you may have, using language that demonstrates you need clarification. Thus, you may need to say:

- "Please explain this to me."
- "I don't understand this research."
- "I have some information I would like to share."
- "I would like to get a second opinion."
- "I would like to do more research or take more time before making my decision."

Who Decides if You Have a Cesarean Section?

As mentioned above, the bill of rights deems you have the legal right to refuse a cesarean, even if the decision may result in the death of you or your baby. What happens, however, if you want a c-section instead of undergoing a vaginal delivery, even if there are no apparent medical reasons to have one? The answer is that you can choose to have this elective procedure.

However, it is crucial to keep in mind that a cesarean delivery is major abdominal surgery, and it has its share of risks. During a vaginal delivery, the muscles you use are more likely to squeeze out the fluid from your baby's lungs, thus making breathing issues less likely. This mechanism is absent in a cesarean birth, so it increases the likelihood of a baby having breathing difficulties and requiring neonatal care (Jones, n.d.). Moreover, it takes around six weeks to completely recover from this surgical procedure.

If you opt for a c-section, you will usually be advised to meet with your OB-GYN team to discuss your reasons for the choice. If you have a phobia of childbirth, counseling may be recommended to overcome your anxieties.

TYPES OF BIRTH

Physiologic (Natural) Birth

Physiologic or natural birth proponents deem this type of labor inherently safer and healthier because no unnecessary interventions disrupt the normal physiological processes (Birth Tools, n.d.). This type of delivery is characterized by the spontaneous commencement and progression of labor, vaginal delivery of the baby, physiological blood loss, skin-to-skin contact, keeping you and your baby together during the postpartum period, and supporting early breastfeeding (American College of Nurse-Midwives, 2021).

Factors That Can Interfere With Physiologic Birth

Physiologic childbirth is not the same as natural childbirth since the latter can occur after induction, an episiotomy, and similar procedures. Even with some complications, opting for a physiologic or natural birth can boost the outcomes for you and your baby.

Factors that can interfere with physiologic childbirth include:

- the induction of labor
- time or staffing constraints
- pain medications
- an episiotomy
- cesarean/vacuum/forceps delivery
- early cutting of the umbilical cord before it has stopped pulsating
- separating your and your baby after birth
- restricting food or drink
- any situation in which you feel unsupported or threatened

The Benefits of a Physiologic Birth

Important factors that influence your ability to have a natural birth without intervention include your health and fitness, your knowledge and confidence about birth, your cultural beliefs and what you have been taught about childbirth, having access to healthcare and a support system, and having the chance to make informed decisions alongside your healthcare provider. Having a midwife can be very helpful, as they are experts in helping women have natural, healthy births.

The benefits of a physiologic birth include:

- reduced peripartum death owing to surgical complications
- improved likelihood of breastfeeding, which has immediate and life-long advantages for the baby
- feeling emotionally healthy and powerful
- reduced out-of-pocket costs

- shorter hospital stays and faster recovery times
- smaller chance of major surgery for severe bleeding, scarring, infections, and reactions to anesthesia.

Cesarean Birth

Approximately one in three women in the US has had a cesarean delivery. Moreover, about 26% of women with low-risk pregnancies and full-term babies positioned headfirst, i.e., women who are considered capable of having a healthy vaginal birth, have c-sections (Escobar, 2018).

The reasons for cesarean delivery are many and include:

- prolonged labor
- abnormal fetal positioning
- fetal distress
- cord prolapse
- large baby, narrow pelvis
- previous cesarean delivery
- your health/physical condition

Also, there is no definitive rule for when a c-section is warranted due to a "failure to progress" in labor. As a result, the decision to perform a c-section can vary greatly and depend on an individual doctor's opinion.

The Benefits of a C-Section

The practical benefits of having a c-section include scheduling a birth in advance if it is elective. Sometimes it is deemed necessary—for instance, if the baby is in a feet-first position and the health care professional cannot turn the baby into a head-down position or if the baby is very large and the mother has a narrow pelvis (Nierenberg & Wild, 2021). C-sections are sometimes recommended if labor takes excessively long, the mother has developed signs of infection, or the baby is not getting sufficient oxygen.

Tips for Avoiding a C-Section

If you wish to avoid a c-section, important strategies include:

- Choose a healthcare provider after discussing their c-section rates and policies. Some healthcare providers automatically suggest a c-section if a patient has had a birth via c-section in the past. Others will try for a vaginal delivery first.
- Check the c-section statistics at your hospital. Depending on the hospital, these can vary from 2.4% to 36.5%.
- Hire a doula. They will be an essential advocate during birth. Statistics show women with a doula are 26% less likely to have a c-section (Sheehy, 2020).
- Learn about labor and delivery by taking a birthing course. It is essential to read up on topics such as birthing positions and labor durations and learn interpersonal skills that will help healthcare staff see you as someone they want to support (Escobar, 2018).
- Read informative books. Many useful and fascinating books may inspire you as you consider whether or not a physiologic birth is right for you. These include *Your Best Birth: Know All Your Options, Discover the Natural Choices, and Take Back the Birth Experience* by Ricki Lake and Abby Epstein, *The Birth Partner* by Penny Simkin, and *Natural Childbirth the Bradley Way: Revised Edition* by Susan McCutcheon.
- Access online resources such as:
- **www.kidshealth.org**: for information on birthing centers and hospital maternity services
- **www.americanpregnancy.org**: for resources on birth choices by health care providers
- **www.mana.org**: a website created by the Midwives Alliance of North America.
- **www.betterhealth.vic.gov.au**: for information about pregnancy and birth care options
- **www.everymothercounts.org**: features essential conversations about pregnancy, birth, and beyond

- Learn about CenteringPregnancy, a model of small group care developed by Sharon Rising, CNM. This type of care involves attending regular, provider-led group meetings to address all components of a pregnancy, not just your and your baby's physical health. Classes start at around three months of pregnancy, with groups meeting every two to four weeks for sessions lasting between one and two hours. Topics covered include preparing for giving birth, soothing discomfort, nutrition, breastfeeding, and postpartum contraception (Taylor, 2021). These sessions replace routine clinic visits, during which your provider will check your blood pressure, weight, and other data while listening to any concerns or questions you may have.

CHOOSING THE PLACE OF BIRTH

You can give birth in a hospital, at an out-of-hospital birth center, or at home. Often, this choice depends on factors like your culture and philosophy of birth, the preferred type of care a provider can give, and the number and type of caregivers accessible to a patient (Childbirth Connection, n.d.). Make sure the place of birth you choose offers the following:

- care based on evidence about safe and effective practices
- a setting that will support your body's natural ability to give birth if you opt for a natural or physiologic delivery
- staff are deeply committed to making you feel supported and cared for
- personalized care depending on your health needs, values, and preferences

It is important to contact your insurance company to ask if your plan covers your preferred setting and care provider. You should ask about the coverage offered for any elective services you may require, such as the assistance of a doula.

What Are the Advantages of a Home Birth vs. A Hospital Birth?

The percentage of out-of-hospital births in the US stands at around 1.61%. However, the popularity of home births has increased considerably over the years. From 2004 to 2017, they increased by 77% (MacDorman & Declerq, 2018). Some of the benefits of home delivery include:

- giving birth in a private, familiar environment surrounded by loved ones, including other children
- ability to deliver a baby naturally with previously purchased aids such as a pool, bathtub, birthing ball, or something similar
- having a midwife deliver the baby in a freer setting
- cultural and religious benefits

If you choose to have a home birth, you should create a backup plan with your midwife. The midwife will monitor labor progress closely and is ready to transfer you to a hospital if required.

Generally, giving birth at home costs one-half to one-third of the cost of a hospital delivery. Unfortunately, if this type of delivery is not covered, out-of-pocket expenses can be so costly that they are prohibitive. Sometimes a lack of insurance or Medicaid coverage stops women from having an out-of-hospital birth.

The advantages of a hospital birth include proximity to emergency services, having the support of a nursing team, and receiving a c-section quickly if necessary. On the downside, your birthing positions may be limited, and the number of support people allowed in the delivery room may be limited. You may not be able to have the type of birth you wish, such as a water birth. Finally, your doctor may be unavailable during the delivery time (MedicineNet, 2021). Having a midwife or doula on hand can help, as they can clear their schedule closer to your delivery date.

CHOOSING A HEALTHCARE PROVIDER

When giving birth, you can choose to be attended to by a physician or a midwife. Midwives can be part of a care team at a hospital or take charge of a home delivery. There are five types of midwives (Graduate Nursing, n.d.). They are:

- **Certified Nurse-Midwives (CNM) and Certified Midwives (CM)**: These midwives are highly trained health care professionals who care for women through all life stages— from adolescence through menopause. They provide well-woman care, birth control, pregnancy care, childbirth care, and care during the postpartum period. While CNMs are nurses and CMs are not, both have completed a graduate-level nursing degree and passed a certification exam from the American Midwifery Certification Board.
- **Certified Professional Midwives (CPM)**: These midwives are certified by the North American Registry of Midwives and have passed the NARM exam. They monitor a mother's wellbeing from the prenatal to postnatal stages; refer women to an obstetrician if required; provide mothers with individualized care, information, and support; and use as few technological interventions as possible.
- **Direct-Entry Midwives**: These midwives specialize in home births and free-standing births. No national certification or licensing is available. However, each state has applicable legal requirements covering the position. A Certified Professional Midwife, Certified Midwife, or Certified Nurse-Midwife can be a direct-entry midwife. Some states require them to hold specific certifications, while others do not. Most direct-entry midwives are self-employed.
- **Lay Midwives**: These midwives are uncertified or unlicensed and often have an informal education in the field. Some states require licensing for this type of midwife; others do not.

What Is the Difference Between a Doula and a Midwife?

The main difference between a doula and a midwife is that a doula provides physical and emotional support during labor and aids you in a non-medical capacity. On the other hand, a midwife is a qualified professional who can help you deliver your baby, identify complications in both you and your baby, access medical assistance, and carry out emergency measures.

Doulas help educate women about their choices and can provide assistance during labor, childbirth, and the postpartum stage. They obtain their certification from Childbirth International, D.O.N.A (Doulas of North America), and the Childbirth and Postpartum Professional Association (C.A.P.P.A.).

CHAPTER SUMMARY

After reading this chapter, you probably feel like you have tons of information to consider. Take this time to read everything you can about birth, and remember to:

- Know your rights.
- Make informed, evidence-based decisions.
- Know you can refuse interventions you do not desire.
- Consider the best place for your delivery.
- Choose the right health care provider and consider a midwife or doula if you choose to have a hospital delivery.
- Weigh the pros and cons of a vaginal or c-section delivery.

In addition to making important decisions regarding the birth, taking care of yourself in the months leading up to the big day is vital. Ch Three offers advice for staying healthy during pregnancy.

PART II

Self-care during pregnancy is the first gift that the mother can give to her child.

— MARY THOMPSON

The best advice for a healthy pregnancy is to take care of yourself. Self-care during pregnancy is critical to your and your baby's overall health and well-being. It promotes your physical and emotional well-being. It ensures you're getting the sleep, rest, and restorative activities you need to stay healthy, alert, and energized. Self-care includes taking care of yourself emotionally. It can be as simple as taking time out to relax with a massage or a cup of tea, or discussing your feelings with a trusted friend or therapist.

There is no right way to care for yourself during pregnancy. You are the best judge of your needs and what you can handle. Pregnancy is a period of physical, emotional, and social changes, which can sometimes be overwhelming. The important thing is to take care of yourself throughout your pregnancy to provide the best possible environment for your baby to grow and thrive.

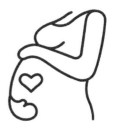

TAKING CARE OF YOUR HEALTH DURING PREGNANCY

P regnancy is a unique opportunity for you to harness the many benefits of healthy living and kickstart a lifestyle that can put you in good stead even after your baby is born. Florence was a confessed fast food and sugar addict. She was a little distressed about switching to a healthier diet but discovered (shout-out to celebrity chef Jamie Oliver) healthy meals could be delicious—even more so than her favorite fast foods. She was surprised to learn they could be comforting, serving as soul food.

Moreover, a great meal takes as little as 15 minutes or half an hour to prepare. Florence slowly began preparing more and more meals at home. She continues to make tasty meals for her family and friends.

FOODS TO ENJOY AND FOODS TO AVOID DURING YOUR PREGNANCY

The old saying "you're eating for two" is technically correct. Still, you only need to consume around 300 more calories per day, especially in the latter months of your pregnancy when your baby is bigger (Kids Health, n.d.). However, suppose you have a very low BMI. In that case, your health provider may recommend consuming more calories, so obtaining a custom nutritional plan can be helpful.

Eating well during pregnancy isn't very complicated. It involves eating a variety of foods while following recommended dietary guidelines. These include lean meats and other protein sources; Omega-3- and vitamin D-rich fatty fish like salmon, fiber-rich fruits and vegetables, whole-grain bread, and low-fat dairy products. Legumes such as lentils, peas, chickpeas, and beans are excellent sources of nutrients such as protein, calcium, fiber, iron, and folate. Calcium, which strengthens bones and is vital in pregnancy, is found in dairy products, broccoli, and kale.

You should drink several glasses of water daily to maintain optimal hydration.

Food and beverages to avoid include:

- high-mercury fish (swordfish, king mackerel, bigeye tuna, tilefish from the Mexican gulf, and shark)
- raw fish and shellfish (including sushi and sashimi, ceviche, and raw oysters)
- refrigerated smoked seafood
- undercooked meat, poultry, and eggs
- undercooked luncheon meats and hotdogs
- refrigerated meat spreads and pâtés
- unpasteurized dairy products
- unwashed produce
- excess caffeine—it is recommended that pregnant women consume less than 200mg of coffee a day, a little less than one cup of brewed coffee
- alcohol
- herbal tea—few studies have been carried out on the effects of some herbs on a baby's health

Important Supplements

Your health care provider will most likely recommend supplements to boost levels of critical nutrients like folic acid, iron, and calcium, which are particularly important for you. Ideally, you should consume a minimum of 1,000 mg of calcium, 30 mg of iron, and 400–800 micrograms of folic acid per day.

The embryonic neural tube is formed during the first few weeks of pregnancy and eventually develops into your baby's brain and spinal cord, so if you are planning a pregnancy, speak to your doctor about starting folic acid supplements. Research has shown that taking them one month before and during your first three months of pregnancy can reduce the likelihood of neural tube defects, such as spina bifida.

STAYING ACTIVE DURING YOUR PREGNANCY

Exercise during pregnancy has a wide range of benefits. It relieves aches and pains by toning and strengthening the muscles in your thighs, back, and buttocks. Boosting your cardiovascular fitness can make your pregnancy and delivery easier. It can increase your endurance and improve your controlled breathing techniques, which are very handy during a long delivery. Exercise can help you gain less fat, though you should not aim to lose weight during this time. Instead, the main priority should be to maintain a good fitness level.

Spanish researchers (Perales et al., 2017) have found the percentage of women who meet exercise recommendations during pregnancy is low, primarily because of their confusion about the type of exercise to undertake. Ask your doctor to suggest suitable activities. Leading an unhealthy, inactive lifestyle during pregnancy can increase your risk of weight gain, gestational diabetes, lower back pain, urinary incontinence, and pre-eclampsia. It can also increase your risk of having a c-section.

Exercise can save your baby from health problems when they are adults. A lab study undertaken by scientists at the University of Virginia Health System (Laker, 2020) has shown exercise prevents the transmission of metabolic diseases from an obese parent to a child. These findings clearly show exercise is an important preventive measure that merits the time and effort involved.

Factors That Can Affect Your Routine

You may need to limit your exercise if you have pregnancy-related high blood pressure, early contractions, bleeding, or a premature amniotic sac rupture. It is always important to speak to your health care provider before beginning a new routine or even continuing one you are used to.

Beneficial Activities During Pregnancy

After receiving approval from your healthcare provider, you may enjoy trying the following activities, in addition to traditional favorites such as walking and swimming:

- **Yoga:** Numerous studies have established the many benefits yoga can offer you. These include stress reduction and a reduced chance of anxiety and depression (Newham et al., 2014), and improved heart health for your baby after birth (Science Daily, 2011).
- **Stretching**: Stretching exercises can reduce the risk of pre-eclampsia (pregnancy-induced hypertension) more effectively than walking (Science Daily, 2008).
- **Resistance Exercise**: Moderate resistance exercise can soothe common pregnancy symptoms and improve your sense of control, as found by research from the Sahlgrenska Academy (Science Daily, 2015).
- **Pilates**: A 2021 study (Ghandali et al.) found Pilates exercise during pregnancy significantly reduced labor pain intensity and the length of the active phase of labor while increasing satisfaction with the labor process.

You may want to run many more activities by your caregiver, including low-intensity dance aerobics, stationary bike riding, and weight training. Your health provider should indicate limits on weight training.

MAINTAINING YOUR BACK HEALTH

Back pain during pregnancy affects between 50% and 80% of women (Cedars Sinai, n.d.). For 10% of women, the pain can be so severe that it interferes with their ability to carry out everyday activities. The cause of the pain can be hormonal, since increased hormone release will cause the ligaments to soften and the joints to loosen in the pelvic area in preparation for labor. However, pain can be attributed to additional weight, poor posture, a shift in your center of gravity, or stress.

Lower back pain usually arises between the fifth and seventh months of pregnancy. For some, it can begin when they are just two months into their pregnancy.

Pain can be most substantial in the lumbar area, just above the waist, and in the middle back. It can radiate down towards the leg or foot and be felt in the back of the pelvis, below the waist, across the tailbone, or on just one side.

To relieve back pain, try the following:

- Maintain good posture while you are sitting and standing. Invest in good, ergonomic furniture that supports your back and has an adjustable height so your feet are flat on the floor.
- When exercising, opt for workouts that strengthen your back and abdominals. Pelvic tilts are highly recommended to prevent back pain. They involve lying on the floor with your knees bent and your feet flat on the floor and gently tilting your pelvis and hips backward so the curve of your back is flat on the floor. When trying this exercise out, maintain the tilted posture for a few seconds, lengthening the amount of time as you become accustomed to it.
- Try taking a warm bath, having a pregnancy massage (after the first trimester), and wearing supportive shoes.

Acupuncture can help soothe back pain during pregnancy, as can chiropractic care.

- Avoid heavy lifting and any activities that involve climbing ladders, walking up steep hills, bending, or twisting, as these could affect your back.
- Aim to sleep on your side. Many women use maternity pillows that are long and curved to provide extra support.

SEX DURING PREGNANCY

You can continue to have sex throughout your pregnancy unless your caregiver recommends otherwise. You may find an increase in sensitivity owing to increased blood flow to your breasts, sexual organs, and vulva. Neither vaginal sex nor orgasms can cause damage since your uterine muscles and amniotic fluid safely protect your baby. A mucus plug develops around the cervix, offering additional protection (Medical News Today, n.d.).

In the later stages of pregnancy, orgasms or sexual penetration can trigger Braxton-Hicks contractions. These are mild, harmless contractions of the uterus that tone the muscles in your uterus and help prepare the cervix for birth (Pregnancy, Birth, and Baby, n.d.). These contractions appear irregularly, and they can last for about 30 seconds. Regular labor contractions last longer—generally, from 30 to 70 seconds.

Which Sex Positions Are Best During Pregnancy?

You should generally choose a comfortable position for yourself, avoiding any position that puts pressure on your belly as you enter the later stages of your pregnancy. The missionary position, for instance, can compress blood flow to you and your baby, particularly after Week 20.

Positions you may find amenable include sex from behind, being on top of your partner, spooning, side-by-side sex (similar to spooning except you are facing your partner), the reverse cowgirl, standing, and sitting. Some women may enjoy anal sex. If you opt for anal sex, be vigilant about any body parts, including fingers, passing from the anus to the vagina. This can spread bacteria and result in infection.

When having sex, you may want to avoid deep penetration in the later stages of pregnancy, especially the third trimester, to avoid irritating the cervix (Shinn, n.d.). This is simply because increased blood flow during pregnancy can make the cervix bleed anytime something comes in contact with it. Bleeding sometimes occurs during sex, a vaginal ultrasound, or a Pap smear test. This type of bleeding is not considered a threat to you or your baby (Ariela, 2021).

Finally, oral sex is always an alternative to penetrative sex.

A word of warning: if you are having oral sex, your partner should never blow air into your vagina since doing so can cause a blood vessel blockage by an air bubble. This can be fatal for you or your baby.

GETTING A GOOD NIGHT'S SLEEP

Progesterone levels increase when you are pregnant, and your metabolism increases by up to 20%. This can make you feel sleepy and tired in the daytime. Aim to stick to a good sleeping routine, obtaining eight to ten hours of sleep at night. Remember, sleep quality is as important as sleep quantity (Suni, 2021). The Sleep Foundation defines good sleep quality as:

- falling asleep quickly within 30 minutes of getting into bed
- sleeping the whole night through, waking up no more than once
- being awake for no longer than 20 minutes once you have fallen asleep

What Sleep Disorders Can Occur During Pregnancy?

The Sleep Foundation reports (Pacheco, 2022) that about 50% of women have insomnia during pregnancy due to shifting hormone levels, physical discomfort, and excitement or anxiety about the upcoming birth. Factors such as breast tenderness, an increased heart rate, shortness of breath, a higher body temperature, leg cramps, and waking frequently to urinate can make it harder to get good quality sleep.

You may have specific sleep disorders such as:

- obstructive sleep apnea, which manifests itself as snoring and lapses in breathing
- restless leg syndrome, an unstoppable urge to move the legs
- gastroesophageal reflux disorder, commonly known as heartburn, feeling like a burning sensation in the esophagus, especially when lying down. GERD affects up to 25% of women in the first trimester and up to 50% of those in their last trimester.

If you have one of these disorders, speak to your health provider, as there are specific treatments for each issue. For instance, you can use a continuous positive airway pressure device (CPAP) for obstructive sleep apnea, and antacids may help soothe GERD. You may use massage, supplementation, or heat therapy for leg restlessness and pain.

To help you enjoy a good night's sleep, follow these tips:

- Keeping your room at a cool temperature will help you feel sleepy. 60°F is ideal.
- Avoid using screens in the hours leading up to bedtime, as these can increase alertness.
- Sleep in a comfortable bed. If you are shopping for a new mattress, choose one with good back support, temperature regulation, cooling abilities, and the ability to support your body's pressure points.
- Invest in blackout curtains and soundproofing. Distractions such as noise and light can keep you tossing and turning.

- Don't overdo your power naps. Limit their duration to 20 or 30 minutes. If you sleep longer, you may find it hard to fall asleep at night.
- Use a maternity pillow for extra support.
- Sleep on your side instead of your back.
- Avoid midnight snacking.

MAINTAINING GOOD DENTAL HEALTH

Pregnancy can increase the risk of health issues leading to complications. There is a link, for instance, between gum disease and giving birth to a premature baby. You should know how pregnancy can indirectly cause health problems (March of Dimes, 2019). Something seemingly unimportant like tiredness can lead you to brush your teeth less frequently, causing plaque buildup on your teeth and along the gumline.

If you develop cavities, the bacteria in your mouth can pass infection to your baby. Pregnancy can cause your teeth to become loose. Rising progesterone and estrogen levels can temporarily loosen the bones and tissues that keep teeth firmly in place. Finally, acid can erode your tooth enamel if you vomit excessively from morning sickness, leaving your teeth more vulnerable to decay.

During pregnancy, you may develop lumps on your gums that appear red. These are called "pregnancy tumors." They are harmless and disappear after delivery.

Prioritizing your dental health and keeping dental checkup appointments is vital throughout your pregnancy. Early detection of cavities can enable your dentist to take action quickly without the need for complex procedures that require sedation or general anesthesia, which, in some cases, could be harmful to your baby.

Small cavities usually require local anesthesia, which is safe during pregnancy (Cards Dental, 2019). Pain relievers, antibiotics, and dental X-rays are considered safe. Still, you should always let your dentist know you are pregnant to take the safest option.

Exercise good oral hygiene by brushing your teeth twice a day and flossing once. Floss before you brush to aid in plaque removal. (Horbar, 2020).

AVOIDING HARMFUL SUBSTANCES

Make it a point to avoid alcohol, cigarettes, vaping products, and other drugs, as they may lead to congenital abnormalities, as can certain medications, including some anti-cancer drugs, some anti-epileptic drugs, warfarin, some tranquilizers, some selective serotonin reuptake inhibitors (SSRIs), hormones like androgens and progestins, and more. The list of chemicals and medications to avoid is long, so reporting everything you have been taking to your physician is one of the most critical steps to take during your pregnancy (Sick Kids Staff, n.d.).

Which Medications Should You Avoid During Pregnancy?

If you were taking prescription medications before becoming pregnant, ask your healthcare provider if you can safely continue taking them during your pregnancy. Inquire about over-the-counter medications as well—although most have a good safety profile, they may be dangerous during particular stages of your pregnancy.

You can take acetaminophen for fever, headaches, or pain. If you take this medication, aim to do so for a short duration only. There is a link between using this medication for 28 days or longer and your baby's higher risk of developmental delays, autism, and ADHD (National Institutes of Health, 2019). Taking acetaminophen frequently during the second half of pregnancy can increase a baby's chances of having asthma.

Meanwhile, NSAIDs—non-steroidal anti-inflammatory drugs such as Ibuprofen—are linked to a higher likelihood of heart or gastrointestinal problems in babies. They are not recommended during the final trimester of pregnancy because they can cause high blood pressure in a baby's lungs.

Other medications that cause problems include opioids, including oxycodone, morphine, and codeine, which can lead to heart problems for your baby and premature birth, preterm labor, or stillbirth.

As a general rule, do not take any medication without first consulting with your doctor. If you have ever used illegal drugs or have an addiction to alcohol or any substance, get treatment from your healthcare provider. Do not try to do it alone, as quitting suddenly can cause severe issues. Your doctor can prescribe medications to help you gradually reduce your dependence on drugs (Cleveland Clinic, n.d.).

WORKING DURING YOUR PREGNANCY

If you work outside the home, you may wonder how to inform your boss and colleagues of your news. Some mothers wait for the first trimester to pass before sharing the news, as the risk of miscarriage is lower. Others may want to wait longer—for instance, if they are awaiting amniocentesis results. Whenever the time feels right for you, inform your boss of the time you may need off for prenatal care visits, offering to make up time if necessary. You can ask to change your role at work if it involves significant physical effort or exposure to chemicals that can potentially be dangerous for your baby.

Thinking About Maternity Leave

The Family and Medical Leave Act of 1993 (FMLA) grants 12 weeks of unpaid leave annually for mothers of newborns or newly adopted children, provided they work for a company with 50 or more employees. Some states extend this right to women working in companies with fewer than 50 employees. To be eligible for this leave, you must have worked for your employer for at least 12 months and worked at least 1,250 hours over the previous 12 months.

Conditions can vary greatly from company to company. Some employers offer paid maternity leave. It is important to ask a knowledgeable human resources person at work if they can inform you of what rights you have and what type of medical care your health insurance covers. Sometimes, you may need to change your plan to ensure your baby has coverage. You should find out if there are any services or options available that can be of use. These can include flex-time, working from home, and having a private space at work where you can pump breast milk.

WILL YOUR PREGNANCY AFFECT YOUR TRAVEL PLANS?

If you had a trip booked before discovering you were pregnant, know that, in most cases, it is perfectly safe to travel until you are close to your due date. Your health care provider will let you know if there are any reasons why it might be best not to travel. They may advise you against traveling, for instance, if you have had health conditions or complications such as preeclampsia, prelabor rupture of membranes, or preterm labor.

Generally, the optimal time to travel is between Weeks 14 and 28 (The American College of Obstetricians and Gynecologists, n.d.). During this stage of your pregnancy, your morning sickness may be over, and you may still feel able and energetic enough to get around. Most airlines allow pregnant women to fly within the United States until around Week 36 of their pregnancy. You must contact your airline for international flights since cut-off times may differ.

Having a checkup before you leave is advised and ensures your vaccines are up to date. If you have any symptoms of health issues, including bleeding, vomiting, diarrhea, pelvic pain, or any worrisome signs during your travels, seek emergency help immediately.

When traveling by plane, get up from your seat frequently to stretch your legs and get your circulation going. Avoid carbonated drinks, and book an aisle seat so you can get up as often as you like.

PREGNANCY AND PETS

Pets are beloved members of many American families. Two out of every three homes have a pet, and some 393.3 million pets live in the US (Spots, 2022). If you have a pet or are thinking of getting one, you may wonder if caring for a pet can carry health risks. Dogs are generally safe to have around at this time, but you need to ensure your pup is well-trained so he doesn't jump up on your belly or gnaw and bite. Behavioral training will come in handy when your baby arrives. Make sure your pets are up to date with vaccinations as well.

Caring for Cats

Doctors generally advise being careful when handling cats during pregnancy, as they may carry toxoplasmosis, an infection caught by a parasite that is passed through a cat's feces. Cats can get this infection if they spend time outside or go hunting. Toxoplasmosis can be passed to you when you clean your cat's litter tray, touch soil or other surfaces where your cat may have been, or consume undercooked meat (March of Dimes, 2019). To prevent infection, ask a non-pregnant family member to perform kitty litter duties, keep your cat indoors, wash your hands after gardening, or ask someone else to perform gardening duties. Feed your cat canned or dried food. Avoid feeding them undercooked meat.

Other Pets

Other pets that may pose a risk during pregnancy are rodents, which could carry a virus called lymphocytic choriomeningitis, or LCMV. This virus can cause miscarriages and severe birth defects. If you have these pets, ask a family member to clean their cage, wash your hands with soap and water if you have handled them, and keep them in a separate part of your home.

Snakes, lizards, frogs, turtles, reptiles, and amphibians can cause bacterial infections like salmonellosis and listeriosis. These infections can cause preterm labor, miscarriage, stillbirth, and fatal infections in newborns. Doctors usually advise pregnant women to avoid having this type of animal at home during pregnancy.

CHAPTER SUMMARY

For a safe and hassle-free pregnancy, make sure to:

- Eat a wide variety of healthy, non-processed foods.

- Exercise regularly after running your proposed workout by your health provider.
- Make good sleep quality a priority.
- Take good care of your oral health.
- Discuss any prescribed medications with your health provider.
- Consider how your work arrangements may need to change over the next few months and think about maternity leave.
- Take recommended precautions if you have pets.

Now that you are confidently taking care of yourself, you probably wonder what concerns or discomforts may arise during pregnancy. Chapter Four will discuss some of the most common, including fatigue, constipation, and vivid dreams.

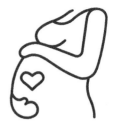

4

COMMON CONCERNS AND DISCOMFORTS

As your pregnancy progresses, you may notice a host of changes, some of which may cause discomfort or worry. When you read about the reasons for the array of new emotions, sensations, and physical changes you may encounter, make a point to be mindful instead of afraid. This chapter will take you through a few concerns and discomforts you may develop along the way. Each pregnancy is unique, and issues that may arise during one pregnancy may not arise in the next.

BREAST TENDERNESS AND OTHER CHANGES

Sore nipples and tender breasts are typical signs of early pregnancy. They occur because of rising progesterone, estrogen, and prolactin levels, a hormone associated with lactation. Other normal changes you may observe include:

- soreness and tenderness
- increased size and fullness
- darkening of the areola
- more visible veins

- colostrum (pre-milk) leaking from the nipples

You can do some things to help ease the discomfort, such as wearing a supportive bra and using a cold compress. If you are concerned about changes in your breasts, please consult your healthcare provider.

CONSTIPATION

Sudden constipation during pregnancy can be uncomfortable if you always have regular bowel movements. Constipation during pregnancy generally occurs because of the rise in progesterone hormones that relax the intestinal muscles, causing food to move through your digestive system slower (American Pregnancy, n.d.). Iron tablets can exacerbate the issue since iron can affect gut bacteria, causing additional problems like gas and bloating (Tolkien et al., 2015).

To prevent or tackle constipation:

- Consume a high-fiber diet, obtaining between 25 and 30 grams of dietary fiber from fruits and vegetables, bran, and breakfast cereals.
- Consume probiotics to help repopulate healthy gut bacteria. Foods high in probiotics include kimchi, yogurt, and kefir.
- Drink plenty of water so your stool is softened.
- Obtain the recommended amount of daily exercise so your digestive system works optimally.
- If you are taking iron supplements, consider taking smaller doses throughout the day instead of one or two large ones.
- If problems persist, ask your doctor to recommend a gentle stool softener.
- See your doctor if you have stomach pain, constipation that lasts longer than a week, bleeding from the rectum, or any other symptoms that worry you.

DREAMS

Vivid dreams and nightmares can arise more frequently during pregnancy. Many pregnant women report having clearer and more detailed dream recollections (Pacheco, 2022). Some mothers dream about meeting their babies or discovering their genders, while others may dream about labor itself. The exact cause of this phenomenon is unknown, though it is thought to be partially related to hormonal changes.

Interestingly, expectant fathers or partners can also dream vividly during this time, and mothers can continue doing so even after the birth of their child.

As you get closer to your due date, your dreams may become more frequent or intense. Dreaming is most likely the body's way of assimilating the array of thoughts and emotions that can race through your mind during this special time in your life. If you feel that dreams affect your mood, take extra care of your sleep routine and try controlled breathing or pregnancy yoga to calm down before bedtime. Occasional nightmares are common. However, if you have frequent nightmares that impact your sleep quality, consider speaking to your health provider or therapist. They may ask you to keep a sleep diary, recording information about your dreams and how they impact your sleep.

FATIGUE DURING PREGNANCY

Feeling tired and sleepy during your first trimester is common during pregnancy. During this time, hormonal changes cause your body to produce more blood to bring nutrients to your baby. At the same time, your blood sugar and blood pressure drop. Higher progesterone levels can make you sleepy, causing a strong urge to rest or nap.

During the second trimester, you may feel a surge of energy. Generally, fatigue is reduced when the placenta is fully functioning. This is a great time to start preparing for the baby's arrival by designing your nursery and stocking up on essentials such as baby clothing.

During the third trimester, fatigue can return. By this time, your baby will be larger, and you may need to urinate more often at night. It may be harder to find a comfortable sleeping position. To cope with exhaustion, ease up on your schedule if you feel drained by too many obligations. Rest as much as possible and prioritize a healthy diet and moderate exercise.

There are a few things you can do to help treat fatigue in pregnancy:

- Get plenty of rest: This may seem like a no-brainer, but getting as much rest as possible when pregnant is essential. Fatigue is often caused by a lack of sleep, so get 8–10 hours of sleep every night.
- Eat healthy foods: Eating a nutritious diet will help your body cope with pregnancy fatigue. Make sure to eat plenty of fruits, vegetables, and whole grains.
- Exercise: Exercise can help increase energy levels and reduce fatigue. A moderate amount of exercise is the key; too much can worsen fatigue.
- Relax: Taking time to relax and de-stress daily can help reduce fatigue. Try taking a warm bath, reading a book, or listening to calming music.

Fatigue can sometimes be a medical issue, such as anemia or gestational diabetes. Therefore, if it is one of an array of new symptoms you are experiencing, see your health provider so you can receive any treatment you require.

FREQUENT URINATION

There are many possible causes of frequent urination during pregnancy, including:

- Hormonal changes: Increased levels of estrogen and progesterone can cause the bladder to fill more quickly
- Pressure on the bladder: Your growing baby can put pressure on your bladder

- Increased blood volume: During pregnancy, the blood volume increases

Urinary frequency eases up during the second trimester since the uterus is higher and there is less pressure on the bladder. However, by the third trimester, your baby's growth may result in increased bladder pressure and a repeated need to urinate. You may experience urinary leakage, especially when you laugh, sneeze, cough, or exercise.

If you are experiencing frequent urination, there are a few things you can do to help relieve the symptoms, including:

- Drink fewer fluids before bedtime to help reduce the need to urinate at night.
- Go to the bathroom regularly. Try to go to the bathroom every two to three hours during the day to avoid becoming too full.
- Wear loose clothing: Wearing loose clothing can help reduce pressure on the bladder.
- Do pelvic floor exercises, commonly called Kegels. These exercises can help strengthen the muscles around the bladder and reduce urinary leakage.

Frequent urination is not a cause for worry. Still, if you have a burning sensation when emptying your bladder, your urine appears cloudy or pink, or you have any other symptoms of a UTI, see your health professional. Remember, UTIs can be more common during pregnancy and precipitate preterm labor.

HEADACHES

Headaches during pregnancy are common, and managing them can be challenging, especially during the first trimester when you should avoid many medications. The exact reason for them is unknown, though hormonal changes and changing blood levels may play a role, as can stress, fatigue, and eyestrain. Nasal congestion and a runny nose can be more common in early pregnancy, which can cause sinus headaches. Finally, low blood sugar levels can trigger headaches, as can caffeine withdrawal if you suddenly give up these beverages during pregnancy.

Migraines can become more prevalent during pregnancy. This type of headache can cause severe pain and throbbing and, in some cases, an aura, light flashes, light sensitivity, nausea, and even vomiting.

There are a few things you can do to help relieve headaches during pregnancy:

- Drink plenty of fluids.
- Avoid known triggers, including cured meats, strong cheeses, and monosodium glutamate (MSG).
- Try placing a cold compress on your forehead for 15 minutes.
- Take over-the-counter pain relievers like acetaminophen, but check with your doctor first to make sure they are safe for you to take.
- Get regular aerobic exercise, which can help to reduce stress and tension headaches.
- Practice relaxation techniques like yoga or meditation.

You can ask your health provider about suitable pain relief. Most pregnant women can safely take acetaminophen for occasional headaches, and your physician may recommend additional safe medications.

If your headache is severe and is accompanied by symptoms such as dizziness or blurry vision, see your health provider. Seek help if severe headaches occur after your 20th week of pregnancy. Migraines can increase the risk of stroke, though the latter is rare. Sometimes, headaches can be related to other problems, including high blood pressure. Seeing your doctor can reduce stress and help put you on the mend.

HEARTBURN

Heartburn during pregnancy is a common complaint. Pregnancy hormones relax the valve between the stomach and esophagus, which can allow stomach acids to back up into the esophagus, causing heartburn.

There are a few things you can do to ease heartburn during pregnancy:

- Eat smaller meals more frequently throughout the day instead of three large meals.
- Avoid trigger foods that make your heartburn worse. Common trigger foods include spicy foods, fatty foods, citrus fruits, tomatoes, chocolate, and caffeine.
- Drink plenty of fluids throughout the day, but avoid drinking during meals.
- Wear loose-fitting clothing to avoid putting pressure on your stomach.
- Sleep with your head elevated to prevent acid from rising in your throat.
- Try over-the-counter antacids to neutralize stomach acids.

If your heartburn is severe and is not relieved by home remedies, you may need to talk to your doctor about prescription medication options.

Heartburn can worsen in your late months of pregnancy when the uterus presses against the stomach.

HEMORRHOIDS

Hemorrhoids can appear at any time during your pregnancy, though for most women, they start at around Week 28. They can be attributed to increased blood flow to the pelvic area and pressure from the growing uterus and baby (Honor Health, n.d.).

Hemorrhoids are common during pregnancy, especially in the third trimester. They are caused by increased pressure on the veins in your pelvis and can be very painful.

There are a few things you can do to treat hemorrhoids during pregnancy:

- Use a hemorrhoidal cream or ointment to relieve pain and swelling.
- Avoid straining during bowel movements.
- Eat high-fiber foods to soften your stool and reduce constipation.
- Drink plenty of fluids to stay hydrated.
- Soak in a tub of warm water for 10–15 minutes a few times a day.
- Apply an ice pack to the area for 10-15 minutes a few times a day.

If home treatment does not improve your symptoms, or if you have large hemorrhoids, you may need to see a doctor for further treatment.

INCREASED VAGINAL DISCHARGE

Vaginal discharge during pregnancy is a normal and common symptom. Discharge occurs when the body produces more mucus to protect the growing baby. This increased mucus production can lead to an increase in vaginal discharge.

In general, there are a few things you can do to help reduce the amount of vaginal discharge you're experiencing:

- Wear loose-fitting, breathable clothing.
- Avoid douching or using vaginal deodorants. Douching can increase your risk of developing an infection.
- Practice good hygiene. Use mild, unscented soap.
- Avoid using scented tampons or pads.

- Drink plenty of fluids to keep your body hydrated. This will help thin out your discharge.
- Eat a healthy diet rich in fruits, vegetables, and whole grains to help boost your immune system.
- Get plenty of rest to help your body to fight off infection.

While some vaginal discharge is expected, some types may indicate an infection. Yeast infections are common during pregnancy because hormone changes affect the vaginal pH. This common yeast infection causes itching, irritation, soreness or stinging during urination, and a cottage cheese-like discharge. If you think you have a yeast infection, tell your health provider about it so you can receive adequate treatment. You should not take antifungal tablets such as fluconazole if you are pregnant or breastfeeding (NHS, n.d.). Ask your healthcare provider if you have any questions or concerns about your medication.

During the last week or so of your pregnancy, you may notice the discharge contains jelly-like pink mucus. This is called a "bloody show." It happens when the mucus plug protecting your cervix from infection dislodges. It is a sign your body is preparing for birth.

ITCHY SKIN

There are a few causes of itchy skin during pregnancy. One possibility is that the skin is stretched and dry due to the expansion of the pregnant belly. This can lead to itching, especially if the skin is already dry or sensitive. Another possibility is that hormones during pregnancy can cause changes in the skin, leading to itchiness. Finally, some women may experience itchiness due to cholestasis, a build-up of bile in the liver that can occur during pregnancy. If you are experiencing itchy skin, talk to your doctor to rule out any serious underlying conditions.

There are a few things you can do to treat itchy skin during pregnancy:

- Use mild, unscented soap when bathing.
- Apply a hypoallergenic moisturizer to your skin after bathing.
- Drink plenty of fluids to stay hydrated.
- Wear loose-fitting clothing made of soft fabrics.
- Avoid scratching the itch, as this can cause further irritation and skin damage.
- Apply a cool compress to the itch if it is particularly bothersome.

Talk to your doctor if the itch is severe or does not go away with home treatment.

LEG CRAMPS

There are a variety of things that can cause leg cramps during pregnancy. The most common cause is simply the increased weight your body is carrying. This extra weight can put a strain on your muscles and nerves, which can lead to cramping. Other causes of leg cramps during pregnancy include dehydration, low levels of potassium or magnesium, and sleeping in an awkward position.

There are a few things you can do to help relieve leg cramps during pregnancy. First, try to avoid standing for long periods of time. If you must stand for a long time, take frequent breaks to move around and stretch your legs. Second, drink plenty of fluids to stay hydrated. Third, eat foods high in potassium and magnesium, such as bananas, leafy greens, and nuts. Finally, if you wake up with a leg cramp, try gently stretching your leg to help relieve the muscle tension. Flex your foot rather than point your toes to get that calf muscle stretched.

There are a few other things you can do to try to relieve leg cramps during pregnancy:

- Stretch your legs before bed.
- Take a warm bath before bed.
- Sleep with a pillow between your legs.
- Exercise regularly.

- Wear comfortable shoes.

MOOD CHANGES

You may experience mood changes during pregnancy due to the changing levels of hormones in your body. You may feel more emotional and weepy, or more anxious or stressed. Other causes of mood changes include lack of sleep, stress, and physical changes. These mood changes are usually most pronounced during the first and third trimesters.

There are a few things you can do to help manage mood changes during pregnancy:

- Get regular exercise. Exercise can help release endorphins, which have mood-boosting properties.
- Eat a healthy diet. Eating a balanced diet can help regulate hormone levels and maintain energy levels.
- Get enough sleep. Sleep deprivation can worsen mood swings. Aim to get at least eight to ten hours of sleep every night.
- Avoid stress. Try to avoid stressful situations as much as possible. If you can't avoid stress, try to find ways to manage it effectively.
- Some self-help techniques can be helpful, such as relaxation and exercise.
- Talk to someone. Talking to a trusted friend or family member about your feelings can be very helpful. You could consider speaking to a counselor or therapist.

Medication may be necessary, but weighing the risks and benefits of any medicine before starting it is essential.

MORNING SICKNESS

Morning sickness is a common symptom during pregnancy and usually starts around the fourth to sixth week. While the cause is unknown, it is believed to be due to the hormonal changes of pregnancy. Morning sickness can occur at any time of the day or night. It is most common during the first trimester, but you may experience it throughout your pregnancy.

Morning sickness is frequently triggered by specific smells, tastes, heat, or excess salivation. Nausea and malaise can be more likely if a mother has similar symptoms from other causes, including migraines, certain smells or tastes, or exposure to estrogen. Women pregnant with twins or other multiples and those who have had morning sickness in past pregnancies can be more likely to experience this issue.

There are several things you can do to help ease morning sickness:

- Get plenty of rest.
- Eat small, frequent meals.
- Avoid strong odors.
- Drink lots of fluids.
- Try ginger in tea or capsules
- Vitamin B6 supplements.
- Wear acupressure wristbands.

Contact your healthcare provider if you find it difficult to keep anything down.

Mild nausea and vomiting usually subside as your pregnancy progresses, so don't let morning sickness worry you. However, if you have severe nausea and vomiting, see your healthcare provider, as this could lead to dehydration, decreased urination, and other problems.

ROUND LIGAMENT PAIN

Round ligament pain is a common, normal pregnancy symptom you may experience during your second trimester. The round ligaments are two strong bands of tissue that attach from the front of the uterus to the groin. As your belly grows during pregnancy, these ligaments must stretch to accommodate your baby. This stretching can sometimes cause sharp, shooting pains on one or both sides of your abdomen or groin.

There are several things you can do to treat round ligament pain:

- Rest when you feel the pain. Take a break and put your feet up.
- Avoid sudden, jerky movements.
- Sleep on your left side, not your back, to take the pressure off your round ligaments.
- Apply heat or ice to the area for 20 minutes at a time.
- Take acetaminophen for pain relief.
- Do gentle stretching exercises throughout the day.
- Wear supportive clothing. A belly band can help support your growing belly and take some strain off your round ligaments.
- Talk to your doctor about pain relief medications. Some over-the-counter options may be safe to take during pregnancy, but you should always check with your doctor first.

SHORTNESS OF BREATH

Most pregnant women experience shortness of breath in the early and late stages of pregnancy due to higher progesterone levels, which cause more rapid breathing. Progesterone expands your lung capacity, allowing your blood to carry large quantities of oxygen to your baby. Later in your pregnancy, shortness of breath can additionally be attributed to your expanding uterus, which takes up more space in your belly and shifts other organs around.

From Weeks 31 to 34, the uterus presses up against your diaphragm. This can make it harder for your lungs to expand, making you feel short of breath. Shortness of breath can improve when you are close to giving birth since, by this time, your baby will move deeper into the pelvis, thus releasing pressure on your diaphragm (March of Dimes, n.d.).

There are several things you can do to treat shortness of breath during pregnancy:

- Take slow, deep breaths.

- Sit up straight and maintain good posture.
- Wear loose, comfortable clothing.
- Avoid hot, humid environments.
- Drink plenty of fluids, especially water.
- Avoid strenuous activity and exercise.
- Get plenty of rest and sleep.
- Try sleeping on your left side to help ease pressure on your lungs

SWOLLEN FINGERS, ANKLES, AND FEET

Swelling during pregnancy is common, especially in the latter part of the term. It is caused by the extra fluid retention that occurs as the baby and uterus grow. Edema can occur in the hands, feet, ankles, and face. Approximately 50% of women report having swollen feet toward the end of their pregnancy. Usually, this worsens at the end of the day and in the later stages of your pregnancy.

Edema occurs because the amount of fluid in your body during pregnancy increases significantly to accommodate your baby (WFMC Health, 2021). To treat swelling:

- Take breaks from standing and sitting.
- Elevate your feet whenever possible. This will help to reduce the pressure on your veins and reduce swelling.
- Drink plenty of water and stay hydrated. This will help to flush out any excess fluid in your body.
- Avoid the heat.
- Lower your sodium intake.
- Wear loose, comfortable clothing. This will allow your skin to breathe.
- Increase your protein intake.
- Get daily light exercise.
- Consider wearing compression socks or leggings for circulatory support.
- Apply a cold compress to the affected area.

See a doctor if you have sudden or significant swelling in your hands, feet, legs, or face. Be wary of pitting edema. You can determine this by pressing down on your skin and seeing if it remains indented. Dizziness, vision changes or blurriness, severe headaches or migraines, difficulty breathing, and abdominal pain are reasons to see your physician.

Be vigilant for painful, warm swelling in one leg, which could indicate deep vein thrombosis (DVT), which is a blood clot in your pelvis or leg (WFMC Health, 2021). Sudden swelling could be a sign of preeclampsia.

UTERINE CRAMPING

Early in pregnancy, it is common to experience mild cramping in your lower abdomen. As your belly grows, you can feel tugging or stretching or a sensation similar to menstrual cramps. Later in pregnancy, you can experience abdominal discomfort as the uterus tightens (Olsson, 2021).

To soothe cramping, rest, a warm bath, deep breathing, staying hydrated, and medication like acetaminophen, if you have your doctor's approval, can help.

Some conditions that cause cramping can be serious. These include:

- ectopic pregnancy–when a fertilized egg implants itself outside of the uterus, commonly in one of the fallopian tubes
- miscarriage
- preeclampsia
- UTI or bladder infection

See your healthcare provider if you are worried or experience severe, regular cramping that worsens over time.

VARICOSE VEINS

Up to 50% of women experience enlargement of the superficial veins in their legs and lower extremities (Penn Medicine, 2018). These veins move blood up the leg, going against gravity to bring blood to the heart. During pregnancy, the growth of the uterus exerts a downward force on venous blood flow, which results in superficial veins growing in size and becoming more visible. These veins can become painful and be accompanied by redness and swelling.

There are several ways to treat varicose veins in pregnancy. Some of the most common methods include:

- Wear compression stockings helps to reduce swelling and discomfort caused by varicose veins. They help to prevent new varicose veins from forming. Purchase high-quality stockings with a minimum strength of 20–30 mmHg. Anything lower may not be helpful, while anything higher may be uncomfortable to wear.
- Elevate your legs to reduce the pooling of blood in your veins. This can help to reduce the pain and swelling associated with varicose veins.
- Regular exercise helps to promote circulation and can help to reduce the symptoms of varicose veins.
- Avoid long periods of standing or sitting. Walking around for a few minutes every hour can help improve circulation and reduce the symptoms of varicose veins.

If you develop varicose veins, point them out to your healthcare professional. These veins are usually harmless, but in rare cases, they can cause severe pain and blood clots. Varicose veins tend to subside a few weeks after your baby is born and fully recover after about a year. If you are concerned about their appearance after this time, there are treatments that can close off the affected veins.

CHAPTER SUMMARY

In this chapter, you learned about some of the most common issues that can arise during pregnancy, including constipation, heartburn, leg cramps, morning sickness, and varicose veins. While most are harmless, some can be a cause for concern, so seeing your doctor may be advisable in some cases.

The Power of Communication

Often, we are too slow to recognize how much and in what ways we can assist each other through sharing such expertise and knowledge.

— OWEN ARTHUR

From 16 weeks on, your baby can hear you in the womb. And it's not just you—they can hear anyone, and they love it! Getting to know voices helps to create a sense of safety and security, and it also benefits their hearing, helping them prepare for the day they'll eventually start talking.

It's easy to think that everything that feeds their development is going on inside you, but the outside world is playing an important role too. Your voice... your partner's voice... the voices of your family and friends... even environmental sounds like music or traffic may be dimly audible as your baby develops.

Your baby is collecting information all the time, information that provides a strong foundation for them to build on when they reach the outside world and continue their development outside of your body.

In a sense, they're on a version of the journey you're on now—collecting information that will serve them throughout the process. Just as you can talk to your baby in the womb to foster this development, you can talk to other new parents to help them collect information, allowing them to make informed choices and approach their pregnancy with confidence.

You can do that right now with just a couple of sentences and a few moments of your time.

By leaving a review of this book on Amazon, you'll let other new parents know where they can find the information that will help feed their sense of security throughout their pregnancy.

By letting new readers know how this book has helped you and what information they'll find within it, you'll show them an easy route to the guidance they're looking for.

Just as you reach out to your developing baby with your voice, you can reach out to other new parents with your words. We're all learning all the time, and that's a beautiful part of the human experience.

Thank you for your support.

Scan QR code for review link.

PART III

Early and consistent prenatal care is the key to a healthy pregnancy.

— COMMON WISDOM

Early and frequent prenatal visits are a must for all pregnant women. Taking the time to see your healthcare provider regularly will help you stay healthy and ensure you have a healthy baby. You can ask questions about your baby's development and get advice on ways to support their growth and development. It will give you peace of mind knowing you are taking the necessary steps to ensure the healthiest possible birth for your baby.

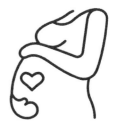

5

THE FIRST TRIMESTER

The first trimester is a period of adjustment. Your most significant psychological challenge of the first trimester is coming to terms with this reality and all it entails.

The first trimester is the most critical period for your baby's development. Your baby's organ systems and physical structure develop throughout this time. Expectant parents frequently keep news of the pregnancy to themselves or close family and friends because birth complications and miscarriages are most frequent during this time.

This chapter will guide you through the wide array of physical and emotional changes you may encounter during your first trimester. You should start prenatal care as soon as you know you are pregnant. In most cases, the first visit will be between Weeks 6 and 8 of pregnancy. You will likely have monthly visits for the first 28 weeks of pregnancy. You will have more frequent visits during the last 12 weeks of pregnancy.

If you have a high-risk pregnancy, you may need to see your health care provider more often. A high-risk pregnancy has certain risks for the mother or baby. These risks may be due to the mother's health, the baby's health, or both.

Prenatal care is provided by obstetricians, family physicians, midwives, and some physician assistants and nurse practitioners. Your doula can accompany you if you wish throughout this period, giving you support and answering questions about the different tests and symptoms you may have.

FETAL GROWTH AND DEVELOPMENT DURING THE FIRST TRIMESTER

Because it usually takes most women at least a month or longer to realize they are pregnant, the first trimester, which is three months long, may seem shorter than it actually is. Although pregnancy lasts 40 weeks, you begin the countdown two weeks before becoming "officially" pregnant. This means you're not actually pregnant for the first two weeks of your pregnancy. It's confusing, but not complicated.

Weeks 1 and 2 are when you have your menstrual period and ovulate. Conception occurs in Week 3, and the fertilized egg implants and settles into the uterus in Week 4.

Remember to consider whether the fetal development described in your other research begins at the LMP, as we do here, or at the presumed moment of fertilization two weeks later. In that case, your estimation of what is happening could be off by two weeks.

Month 1

Overview and highlights:

- last menstrual period
- ovulation: the ovary ruptures, releasing the egg. The sperm fertilizes it inside the fallopian tube.
- implantation: the fertilized egg starts to divide and forms a clump of cells (the zygote), which moves to the uterus and burrows into the uterine lining.

- from oocyte to ovum (egg) to zygote
- the zygote becomes a blastocyst, an embryonic disc with no organ development yet
- the blastocyst becomes an embryo
- the neural tube closed by 28 days after conception
- embryonic heart forms and begins beating

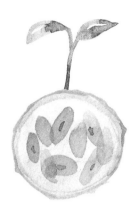

Week 1

This is the first week of your first trimester.

Surprise! You're not pregnant yet. Week 1 begins with your menstrual period. The first day of your last menstrual period (LMP) before becoming pregnant is crucial in determining your anticipated due date and serves as the foundation of your prenatal care plan.

Week 2

Ovulation is assumed to occur on Day 14 of a regular 28-day menstrual cycle. Fertilization occurs in the fallopian tube, creating a new human by the fusion of one ovum, the female egg, and one sperm into one cell, the zygote. The moment of fertilization marks the start of fetal growth and development.

The zygote travels from the fallopian tube to the uterus in three or four days, dividing along the way into 100 or more identical cells. The cells reorganize into a two-layer mass called a blastocyst. The cells in the center will develop into the embryo. The cells on the outside will become the placenta. Throughout your pregnancy, consider the placenta as your baby's main source of nutrition. It delivers oxygen and nutrients to your baby and carries away waste.

The blastocyst will start to burrow into the lush lining of the uterus a day or two later, where it will continue to divide and grow.

Light bleeding that occurs six to twelve days after conception, known as "implantation bleeding," affects 15 to 25 percent of women at this time. Implantation cramps might be experienced.

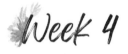 The blastocyst is moving from the fallopian tube and is implanted in the uterine wall. As it continues to grow, a water-tight sac forms around it, gradually filling it with fluid. This is called the amniotic sac, and it helps cushion the growing blastocyst.

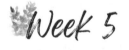 The blastocyst is now officially an embryo. About four weeks have passed since the start of your most recent period. You might be able to get a positive result on a home pregnancy test around this time, which is when your next period would typically be due.

The embryo is undergoing rapid cell division and differentiation. Your tiny embryo is made up of two layers called the hypoblast and the epiblast, from which all of the organs will start to form over the course of the next six weeks. Avoid alcohol, smoking, drug use, and dangerous chemicals, as your baby will be most susceptible to anything that could impair development during this time.

Your baby is about the size of a poppy seed, with a crown to rump length (CRL) measuring 0.12 inches.

This is the first week of your missed period.

Your small embryo, which resembles a tadpole more than a human, is growing rapidly deep inside your uterus. The ectoderm, mesoderm, and endoderm are the three layers that make up your embryo at this point. These layers later give rise to all of the organs and tissues.

The neural tube, which is beginning to form from the top layer, the **ectoderm**, is where the brain, spinal cord, and nerves of your baby are formed. Skin, hair, nails, mammary and sweat glands, as well as tooth enamel, are developed from this layer.

In the **mesoderm**, or middle layer, the circulatory system starts to develop. This week, the tiny "heart" actually starts to beat and pump blood. Your baby's muscles, cartilage, bones, and subcutaneous tissue will all be formed by the mesoderm.

The lungs, intestines, early urinary system, thyroid, liver, and pancreas will all develop from the third layer, or **endoderm**. The primitive placenta and umbilical cord, which provide your baby with nutrition and oxygen, are already at work.

Your baby is about the size of a sesame seed, with the CRL measuring 0.23 inches.

Month 2

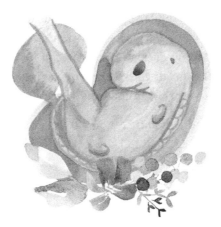

Because crucial structures are developing at this time, err on the side of precaution and avoid harmful substances. Prenatal vitamins with folic acid are crucial to take during this period in order to prevent some birth defects.

Overview and highlights:

- rudimentary heart begins to beat
- the brain, spinal cord, and all other internal organs start to develop
- arm buds form first, then limb buds
- fingers present but not distinct by 10 weeks
- head relatively huge
- embryonic "C" shape
- indentations for the eyes and ears, and lumps for the nose and lips
- tail present
- intestines outside the body

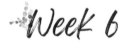 This is a time of rapid growth. The embryo folds into a curved, cylindrical form. Arm buds appear, as well as facial and neck structures. The digestive, urinary, and reproductive systems begin to develop. Her developing eyes and nostrils can be seen as dark spots. On the sides of the head, there are tiny depressions that indicate emerging ears. The vocal cords and tongue are starting to form.

Your baby's arms and legs start out as little paddles that will eventually grow into limbs. A small tail present at the end of the backbone will eventually disappear.

The open neural tube, which eventually becomes her spinal cord and brain, closes up.

The heart is beating 150 times per minute.

Your baby is about the size of a lentil, with the CRL measuring 0.38 inches.

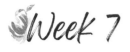 The neural tube is folding in on itself, enclosing the spinal column with the brain at the top. The brain will grow an average of 250,000 cells throughout the entire pregnancy. Due to this rapid development, his head undergoes enormous growth, making it much larger than the rest of his body.

The stomach and esophagus of the embryo begin to develop. The intestines are starting to form.

This week, the lower limb buds will appear and will eventually become his legs. Legs develop nearly a week later than arms since fetal development proceeds from top to bottom.

The cornea, iris, pupil, lens, and retina—the five major components of the eye that enable your baby to see—begin to form this week and will be nearly fully formed in just a few weeks. His eyes are partially covered by developing eyelids.

Your baby has doubled in size since last week, with a tail that will soon vanish.

Your baby is about the size of a blueberry, with the CRL measuring 0.56 inches.

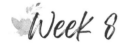 The placenta is functioning normally, and her major organs and body systems are growing. The kidneys are beginning to work, and the intestines are starting to form. The throat and the developing lungs are now connected by airways.

Primitive neural pathways are being created by the branching out of nerve cells. A network of nerves is spreading through your baby's body, making connections not only with each other but with muscles and other tissues, as well as organs like her eyes and ears.

The eyes are now apparent, and the nose and upper lip are formed. Primitive fingers start to emerge in the handpads as her arms and legs go through substantial growth. She starts to develop the eyelid folds and the exterior part of the ear.

Your baby is moving, making small stretches and twitches. These movements begin around seven to eight weeks and can be seen on an ultrasound. It won't be until at least Week 16 that her movements will be strong enough for you to feel.

Your baby is about the size of a kidney bean, with the CRL measuring 0.91 inches.

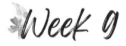 The embryo now has all the necessary body parts, such as elbows and knees. Eyelids have developed and are visible. Parts of the ear are formed and visible, including the ear lobes, but they are not yet in the proper positions. In profile, his nose is visible, but his chin is still unformed.

Primitive toes begin to form, and his paddle-like hands develop fused fingers as his arms and legs continue to grow longer.

The embryonic tail is no longer present.

The heart has formed its four chambers: the left atrium and right atrium are the upper chambers of the heart, and the left ventricle and right ventricle are the lower chambers.

Inside each band of gums, ten tiny tooth buds are forming. The 20 baby teeth that eventually fall out during childhood will develop from them. His teeth begin to harden and attach to the jaw the following week. When your baby gets his first tooth, usually between the ages of four and seven months, you'll start to notice these pearly whites poking out. Although it's uncommon, some newborns are born with teeth.

The embryo can now swallow.

Your baby is about the size of a cherry, with the CRL measuring 1.09 inches.

. . .

Week 10

The embryonic phase comes to an end this week.

All essential internal and external structures are present and have completed the most critical portion of development. She is rapidly growing at this stage in her development, and she has a basic human shape.

The head is still excessively large and makes up about half of her total size. The forehead sits very high on her head and bulges from the rapidly developing brain. The brain is developing at an amazing rate and is starting to make lifelong neural connections. Her limbs and fingers can move because of synapses (nerve impulses) in the spinal cord.

The cornea, iris, pupil, lens, and retina—the major components of the eye that give your infant vision—are all fully developed. Her eyes are covered by eyelids, which are fused shut.

The urogenital system is developing, but the external genitalia are still undefined.

The skin is still translucent. Small details like nails are beginning to form, and her tiny limbs are able to bend.

Your baby is about the size of a strawberry, weighing 0.11 ounces, and CRL measuring 1.38 inches.

~

Month 3

You have most likely started getting prenatal care by the third month.

Your baby's upper body is currently more developed than its lower body at this point, so if you have an ultrasound, you might notice his arms appear longer than his legs.

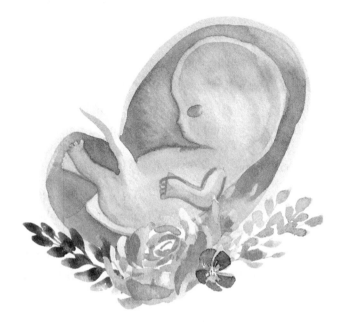

Your risk of miscarriage decreases significantly after three months. This is the time most women feel confident enough in their pregnancy to joyfully announce their good news to anyone who will listen.

Overview and highlights:

- embryo become fetus
- body straightens as the spine and ribs harden
- all internal organs are formed
- intestines in the abdomen
- tail reabsorbed
- external genitals form
- fingers distinct, toes forming
- toenails and fingernails are beginning to grow.
- external ears form
- more distinct eyes, lips, and nose
- tooth buds
- opens and closes his mouth and fists
- swallowing and breathing in amniotic fluid

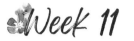 **Week 11**

The embryo is now a fetus.

All her organs are present and functioning. Red blood cells are being produced by the liver, and insulin is being produced by the pancreas.

Your baby kicks, stretches, and even hiccups as her diaphragm develops, but those movements are still too small for you to notice. You probably won't feel your baby move until at least Week 16.

The tiny fingers and toes are now longer and more distinct after losing their webbing.

The blood vessels can still be seen beneath the thin skin, which gives the skin a translucent red appearance.

The sex organs are beginning to develop but are not yet visible on an ultrasound. At this point in her development, she has already started to produce urine.

By the end of this week, the external genitals—the penis and scrotum in boys, the clitoris and labia in girls—will start developing. It will take several more weeks to be able to see the difference between a girl and a boy on an ultrasound.

Your baby is about the size of a fig, weighing 0.29 ounces, and CRL measuring 2 inches.

Week 12

At 12 weeks, your baby is fully formed but highly underdeveloped.

Your uterus has grown to the size of a grapefruit. Your healthcare provider can now feel the top of the uterus (the fundus) low in your abdomen, above your pubic bone. It will be much easier to hear the fetal heartbeat now that it is no longer hidden behind the pubic bone.

Despite the head being noticeably large, about one-third of the CRL, he looks more human than alien at this stage, with unmistakably human facial features. However, the ears are still lower than where they will eventually be.

This week, the reflexes kick in: his fingers will soon begin to open and close; his toes will curl; and his mouth will make sucking movements.

During Week 7, when the stomach and esophagus started to form, the intestines started growing so fast they protruded into the umbilical cord. They will now start to move inside the abdomen as the abdominal wall closes. The anus has begun to develop.

Touchpads are developing on his fingers, which will later become fingerprints.

Your baby is about the size of a plum, weighing 0.49 ounces, and CRL measuring 2.4 inches.

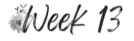 *Week 13*   The fetus has begun recycling the entire volume of amniotic fluid every few hours by swallowing it and eliminating it in urine. Meconium, a greenish-black, sticky substance that builds up in the bowels and becomes your newborn's first poop, is produced by the fetus as it consumes amniotic fluid. Typically, within the first twenty-four hours of birth, babies excrete this substance for the first time. Meconium is passed in utero by up to 10% of fetuses. The fetus could be at risk if they inhale this into their lungs, but generally, it poses no threat. Meconium aspiration is extremely rare, though, as a fetus wouldn't breathe deeply in utero unless they were seriously oxygen-deficient. Healthcare professionals would notice and look into any signs of distress prior to this happening (McCulloch, 2021).

The skin is thin and translucent, but she is beginning to grow a fine, downy hair called lanugo. The whole body will be covered with lanugo by Week 20.

Her fingertips form distinctive ridges that are a key component of her fingerprints.

The skeleton's bones are starting to harden, especially the long bones and the skull. If you're having a girl, her ovaries contain more than 2 million eggs, her lifetime supply.

Your baby is about the size of a pea pod, weighing 0.89 ounces, and CRL measuring 2.8 inches.

Week 14

This is the last week of your first trimester.

The head is large and makes up about one-quarter of the CRL. His eyes are moving toward the front of his face. The nose and taste buds are developing. A small amount of amniotic fluid is ingested and expelled by him as he practices breathing.

As hair follicles begin to form deep within the skin, the skin becomes thicker. These follicles on the chin, upper lip, and eyebrows will begin to produce fine, downy hair around Week 20.

Your baby's facial muscles are contracting in a frown and squint as brain impulses are firing. In addition, he is chewing and sucking. Thumb sucking and the hands opening and closing can be seen on an ultrasound.

The thyroid produces hormones, and the liver produces bile.

Your baby is about the size of a lemon, weighing 1.6 ounces, and CRL measuring 3.15 inches.

MATERNAL BODY CHANGES DURING THE FIRST TRIMESTER

During the first trimester, you may notice the following changes taking place:

- **Morning Sickness:** Despite its name, morning sickness can occur at any time of the day, and it tends to peak around Week 8, lessening by around Week 14. Certain smells or flavors may trigger nausea or vomiting. If morning sickness is severe or sustained and you start feeling dizzy, see your health provider as you may need treatment. Avoid taking over-the-counter medications without consulting your provider first (Cleveland Clinic, n.d.).

- **Increased Appetite and/or Food Cravings:** By around Week 13 or 14, morning sickness will probably be a thing of the past. You may find you start craving specific foods that contain the nutrients you need. While the exact cause of food cravings is unknown, anecdotal evidence does indicate many women experience them. Interestingly, craved foods vary depending on what is regionally and culturally available. For instance, in Tanzania, the most commonly craved food is meat. In contrast, in the US, sweet foods like chocolate, fruits, and juices are more favored during pregnancy (Hainutdzivana et al., 2017).

- **Frequent Urination:** Your growing uterus will start pushing towards your bladder towards the end of the first trimester, making you feel like urinating more often.

- **Expansion of Your Uterus:** Most women don't start showing until they are between 16 and 20 weeks pregnant. However, if you look closely, you may notice a slight protrusion of your belly by Week 13. This is because the uterus expands up over the bony pelvis, and at this point, it reaches the lower abdomen. One of the best things about this is that you may notice you don't need to urinate as frequently as in the early weeks because the pressure on your bladder has lessened.

- **Skin Pigmentation Changes:** Up to 75% of women note changes involving skin pigmentation between Weeks 13 and 27. Commonly called "the mask of pregnancy," these brownish, irregular patches can appear in areas like the forehead, upper lip, and cheeks. They usually disappear after delivery.

- **Dizziness:** Your body works hard to create more blood to support your growing baby, so feeling a little dizzy or lightheaded is normal.

- **Heartburn and Constipation:** As mentioned in Chapter 4, the muscles that help break down food loosen during pregnancy, so food may stay in your stomach a little longer, and you may experience heartburn. Constipation is another nuisance that can be caused by your iron supplement and can be exacerbated by the slower digestion of food.
- **Vaginal Changes:** In Chapter 4, you learned that hormonal changes could cause your breasts to become tender and swollen. Changes can occur in other parts of your body, including the vagina. You may have a thin, white discharge and mild vaginal spotting. Once again, visit the emergency room if you notice the bleeding is heavy or accompanied by pain.

EMOTIONAL CHANGES DURING THE FIRST TRIMESTER

Becoming pregnant can bring both positive and negative emotions. You may be very excited about having a baby but also a little scared, anxious, and awed. It can help to share your feelings with friends and family and talk with your health provider about your concerns, especially if you are feeling depressed or "not like yourself" (Allina Health, n.d.).

Emotional, Educational, and Cultural Matters Are Relevant

You should prioritize the emotional and educational components of your pregnancy. In an article published in *Welfare of Women*, authors Linda Welch and Lisa Miller (2008) remind readers that human communication can be even more critical to women's health than cutting-edge technology. Although significant advances have been made in obstetrics, pregnant women's emotional and educational needs have often been set aside. They deem the need for personalized education and emotional support to be one of the biggest challenges of the 21st century. Power is not to be held by health providers alone but rather shared in an authentic, equal partnership with women. When making health decisions, providers and women should consider the emotional and social consequences of those decisions.

Welch and Miller point out that in current times, pregnancy tends to be treated as an isolated, clinical event. However, it had a deeply religious or spiritual significance in the past. It was celebrated for being an altered or higher physical and psychic state. Families and communities gave extra physical and emotional support. Moreover, before the 20th century, birth was seen as a normal or recurrent part of the female life cycle and a social, family-focused event. It was when women could express their love for and care for other women.

By the 1920s, birth had transformed from a primary female affair to a medically controlled one. Even though modern medicine has significantly reduced maternal and neonatal mortality rates, it has standardized childbirth and created a common birth experience for all women, despite their vast diversity.

Women experience pregnancy on an emotional and physical level. In the beginning, physical issues such as nausea may be predominant. Still, as the moment of birth approaches, anxiety can be the leading cause of concern. Many factors affect your thoughts and emotions and how you cope with them during this special time in your life.

Factors such as whether or not you have given birth before, your socioeconomic status, and the personal support you have are influential. Studies have shown women with high anxiety levels are more likely to experience complications during delivery. Research indicates women who are unconscious during delivery are more likely to have negative beliefs about childbirth.

Welch and Miller cite previous research indicating that for women to have positive pregnancies, they need to accomplish four tasks:

1. Protect herself and her child throughout pregnancy, labor, and delivery
2. Ensure significant people in her life accept her baby
3. Bond with her unknown baby
4. Learn to give of herself

Every task is approached uniquely depending on the individual. This is why health providers should take a personalized approach to pregnancy. A provider's job isn't only to assess physical changes but to discover more about your environment and your capacity to withstand the challenges posed by pregnancy. The provider can start by asking you how you feel about being pregnant, understanding that women often feel ambivalent about having a baby. Joy and stress or anxiety can coexist, and they usually do.

Providers should understand the risks that can contribute to a negative experience. These include having fears of harming the baby, having conflict with one's mother or female family members, and rejecting one's state in the later stages of pregnancy.

You can feel anxious or scared. Your providers should monitor your emotional state, be willing to listen to your partner, if relevant, and understand that women without a support system may be more vulnerable. They should understand how supportive companions can be for women throughout their pregnancy, labor, delivery, and postpartum experience.

Labor support empowers women by putting them, not medical technology, at the center of their birthing experience. Health professionals should provide preconception counseling to women of childbearing age and understand that women's needs and concerns vary from trimester to trimester. Providers should share information verbally and in writing. Birth plans should be encouraged, and women should be encouraged to choose their pediatrician and plan for a one-or two-day stay at their hospital or birth center.

Women should have access to postpartum support—lactation and health consultant visits, support group referrals, and telephone calls to follow up on the new mom's health. The postpartum period can be overwhelming because the changes that occur to a mother's physical and emotional health are dramatic and abrupt. Women are called upon to care for their infants and themselves.

Women who feel supported are better able to bond with their babies. Skin-to-skin contact, touching and looking at the baby, and other actions should be encouraged. Finally, women with babies being cared for in neonatal units should be supported via early psychosocial screening, frequent contact with their primary care provider, and flexible hospital routines.

YOUR FIRST PRENATAL VISIT

It is advisable to schedule your first prenatal visit as soon as you find out you are pregnant. Usually, women have their first prenatal visits around 10 to 12 weeks pregnant. The first visit is the longest, as it will include a thorough medical history, a general physical and gynecologic exam, and routine prenatal lab tests.

Important Questions

During the visit, your provider will ask you questions about:

- you and your family's medical history
- your gynecological history, past pregnancies, and menstrual cycle
- any medication you are taking
- your lifestyle–whether or not you smoke and/or drink alcohol and how much caffeine you consume, if any
- your travel plans, if any, to a place where an infectious disease like malaria, Zika, or tuberculosis may be common
- the date of your last period to calculate your due date, which will be around 40 weeks from the first day of your last period [Mayo Clinic Staff, n.d.]

Let them know if you have any additional information that may be useful to your provider, such as domestic abuse, stress, or past substance abuse.

A Physical Exam

Your provider will check your weight, body mass, and blood pressure. They may perform breast and pelvic exams and screen your thyroid, heart, and lungs. A Pap smear may be taken, depending on how long it has been since your last one.

Routine Prenatal Lab Tests

Your blood type, including your rhesus (Rh factor): The Rh factor is a protein located on the surface of blood cells. If your blood cells have this protein, you are Rh-positive; if they don't, you are Rh-negative. During pregnancy, problems can occur if you are Rh-negative and your baby is Rh-positive. In this case, your body can make antibodies that attack the fetus' blood cells. Treatment can be taken to prevent this from happening (The American College of Obstetricians and Gynecologists, n.d.). If you are Rh-negative, you will be given a RhoGAM injection between Weeks 26 and 28, and then again within 72 hours after delivery to ensure future healthy pregnancies.

Your hemoglobin levels: Hemoglobin is an iron-rich protein found in red blood cells that assists cells in transporting oxygen from your lungs to other parts of your body and carbon dioxide from those parts back to your lungs so it can be expelled. If you have low red blood cell counts or hemoglobin levels, you could have anemia, which will make you feel exhausted. If your blood tests indicate you are anemic, you may need to start taking an iron supplement and/or folic acid supplement in addition to your prenatal vitamins.

Your immunity to certain infections: This includes chickenpox and rubella, unless you have documentation indicating you have been vaccinated against these conditions.

Exposure to other relevant infections: This includes chlamydia and other STDs, HIV, hepatitis B, and more.

You will most likely be asked for a urine sample to test for the presence of protein or sugar, plus any existing bladder infection.

Checking the Fetal Heart Rate

You may hear your baby's heartbeat with a handheld doppler around Week 12. The doctor will apply a little gel and gently slide the device over your belly. You may find hearing your baby's heart rate for the first time very emotional and reassuring.

The Nuchal Translucency Test (NT Scan)

Your doctor may ask to perform the nuchal translucency test to assess the risk of Down syndrome and other genetic disorders. When you are between 11 and 14 weeks pregnant, your baby's neck is still transparent enough that they can measure the amount of clear space in the tissue at the back of the baby's neck. If your baby has more fluid than usual at the back of their neck, it could indicate the presence of a genetic issue.

A sonographer performs this safe and non-invasive scan. They position the sensor over your abdomen so your baby's neck translucency shows. Your baby's chance of having a chromosomal issue is determined by a combination of your age, your baby's gestation age, your blood test results, and the NT scan. A "normal" screening does not guarantee your baby is free of atypical chromosomes. However, it does indicate a problem is unlikely.

Similarly, an "abnormal" result does not mean your baby has a chromosomal problem. It just indicates that it is more likely to have one. Further tests down the line, such as amniocentesis, can determine whether or not this is the case.

Chorionic Villus Sampling (CVS)

Your doctor may recommend chorionic villus sampling (CVS) at some point between Weeks 11 and 14. This test involves taking a small sample of the placenta, which is attached to the uterine wall. It is offered if there is an increased risk of a genetic disorder, including:

- women who will be 35 or older by the expected date of delivery
- family history of specific congenital disabilities
- parental history of a chromosomal abnormality or a genetic disease
- previous abnormal genetic tests or screenings

CHAPTER SUMMARY

Your first trimester is a time of significant change, one in which you may experience fatigue, mood swings, curiosity, and excitement all at once. You can expect to encounter the following during this time:

- bodily changes, including breast growth and, sometimes, the appearance of a small baby bump as your uterus expands and reaches the upper abdomen
- emotional changes, including an enhanced need for support

The first prenatal care visit is the most comprehensive. To get a complete picture of your health, your health provider will take a thorough medical history, perform a physical exam, and collect blood and urine samples.

In the next chapter, you will discover what to expect during your second trimester of pregnancy, including your baby's development and the tests performed during your prenatal visits.

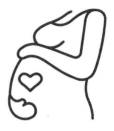

6

THE SECOND TRIMESTER

In the second trimester, which is frequently referred to as the "period of radiant health," you will feel well and largely free from the typical pregnancy discomforts. This middle stage of pregnancy is often regarded as the most enjoyable. By this trimester, morning sickness usually subsides, as do acute fatigue and breast discomfort.

The fetus is about to begin growing in size after finishing the development of all of its organs and systems. As the fetus turns and flips inside the uterus, you might begin to feel movement.

During this trimester, many mothers find out whether their baby will be designated as male or female at birth. This is typically done during an ultrasound that checks physical development at around Week 20.

By this time, you will probably have gathered plenty of information about what to expect in the months ahead. This chapter will focus on how your baby is developing, how you may be changing physically and emotionally, and what tests you will be undergoing from Weeks 13 to 26.

FETAL GROWTH AND DEVELOPMENT DURING THE SECOND TRIMESTER

~

Month 4

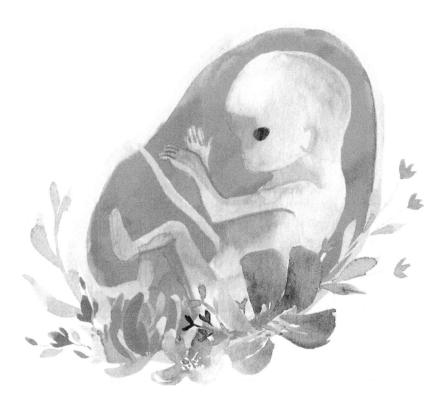

Overview and highlights:

- All internal organs function in some respect
- The nervous system is starting to function
- External genitalia identifiable as boy or girl
- Skin transparent
- Bones form from cartilage

· · ·

- Limbs fully formed
- Eyelids, eyebrows, eyelashes, nails, and hair are formed
- The elbows and knees are actively moving.
- Facial movements, swallowing, yawning, stretching, sucking thumb
- Some sounds are audible
- Movement may be felt

Week 15

This is the first week of your second trimester.

The fetus is continuing to grow and develop at a rapid pace. She is starting to develop more muscles, and the skeleton is starting to harden. The legs are growing longer than the arms. She is actively stretching and moving her limbs.

Your baby's eyelids are still fused shut, but she can sense light. If you shine a bright light on your tummy, she will move away from the beam. Tiny eyebrow hairs are sprouting.

Taste buds are developing in the fetus, and nerves are starting to connect them to the brain. These buds will be fully developed after Week 20.

Your baby is about the size of an apple, weighing 2.7 ounces, and CRL measuring 4 inches.

Week 16

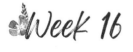

The fetal heart rate ranges between 150 and 180 beats per minute. Depending on where the doctor places the Doppler monitor, you may hear a variety of sounds. A clippity-clop sound, similar to a horse trotting, will be heard if it is directly over the baby's heart. It will sound more like a swoosh-swoosh if the monitor is close to your umbilical cord. Currently, his heart pumps about 25 quarts of blood per day, and this volume will rise.

The eyes are formed and begin to move behind his fused eyelids. The ears are fully formed, functional, and almost in their final position. Your voice and other external noises can be heard by the fetus.

Nerves from the taste buds are forming connections with the brain. He can taste the amniotic fluid he swallows and distinguish between bitter, sour, and sweet flavors. Because the flavors of the foods you eat are absorbed by your amniotic fluid, your baby can start to develop taste preferences.

The head is now more upright and aligned with the body. The upper lip, chin, and eyebrows are starting to grow hair. The hair follicles on the scalp are currently forming a pattern that will last a lifetime. How your baby's hair grows will be determined by this pattern. Babies are born with all the hair follicles they will ever have because new hair follicles don't grow after birth.

Newly developed nerves allow for coordinated movement of the arms and legs.

Between 16 and 22 weeks, you'll begin to feel your baby move, most likely while you are sitting or lying still. The first quiet flutters, or "quickening," are typically detected by seasoned mothers before those who are first-time mothers. Why is it called quickening? The root word, "quick" is an old-fashioned word for "living," as in "the quick and the dead." Therefore, "quicken" means to "achieve the stage of pregnancy at which the child shows signs of life," according to the Oxford English Dictionary.

Your baby is about the size of an avocado, weighing 3.8 ounces, and CRL measuring 4.63 inches.

Week 17

Fetal movements are becoming more coordinated, and she may be able to turn her head. The once-soft cartilage that made up the skeleton is now becoming bone.

The increasing fetal weight is a sign that fat cells are being stored for energy and warmth after birth. These cells appear in areas like the face, neck, and stomach wall, slowly appearing in other body parts over time. The development of sweat glands has begun. The skin layers on your baby will be completely developed by the following week.

The umbilical cord is growing stronger and thicker. It will be about nine inches long and an inch thick at the end of the pregnancy.

Your baby will begin to hear the sounds that are produced by your heartbeat, breathing, and digestion between the ages of 16 and 22 weeks.

Although more common in the 3rd trimester, you might start to feel Braxton-Hicks contractions—those pesky practice contractions. Some doctors and midwives think those contractions help tone the uterine muscle and encourage blood flow to the placenta. They are described as:

- irregular in intensity, typically lasting between 15 and 30 seconds, but occasionally lasting up to two minutes
- infrequent
- erratic
- without a pattern
- they don't get stronger or more frequent
- they diminish until they completely vanish
- more uncomfortable than painful

Your contractions are most likely Braxton-Hicks if they are easing up in any way. These contractions are not deemed "false labor" until you are near your due date.

Your baby is about the size of a turnip, weighing 3.6 ounces, and CRL measuring 5.1 inches.

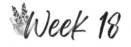 The skull remains soft and flexible to accommodate the rapidly growing brain. Fetal movements are becoming more coordinated, and he may even be able to grasp an object placed in his hand.

The bronchioles, the tiniest tubes in the lungs, begin to form. Alveoli, the respiratory sacs, start to emerge at the ends of these little tubes. These sacs will be filled with tiny blood vessels by the time your baby is born, allowing oxygen and carbon dioxide to flow in and out.

The internal clock that controls the cycle of sleep and waking is developing. The fetus sleeps and awakens periodically throughout the day and may be startled by your movements or loud noises.

Your baby's nerves are developing an internal myelin sheath to protect them. This protective layer develops around nerves, including those in the brain and spinal cord. It is composed of fatty and protein substances. This myelin sheath enables rapid and effective electrical impulse transmission along nerve cells.

An ultrasound clearly shows his lips, nose, and ears. The ears are in their final position, but they still protrude slightly.

The uterus and fallopian tubes have developed and are in their proper positions in girls, and a boy's genitalia are now visible.

Your baby is about the size of a bell pepper, weighing 3.96 ounces, and CRL measuring 5.5 inches.

∾

Month 5

You may start to feel tiny movements this month as your baby develops and becomes more active. Over time, you might start to recognize movement patterns that correspond to waking and sleeping.

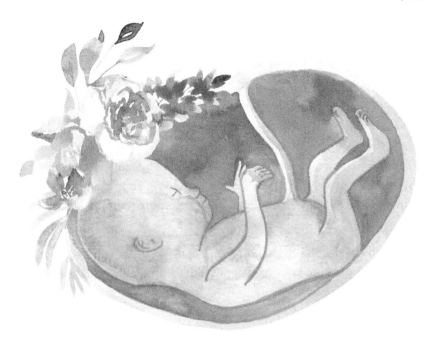

The body of the fetus is covered in lanugo, a fine hair that usually falls out at the end of your baby's first week of life, as well as vernix caseosa, a white waxy coating. It is believed this "cheesy" substance shields her skin from prolonged contact with amniotic fluid. Vernix offers a variety of advantages: It safeguards against harmful bacteria, moisturizes and protects your baby's skin, and promotes the growth of the digestive system and lungs. Just prior to birth, this coating is shed.

Overview and highlights:

- fetal movement is felt
- growth continues with proportions normalizing
- arms and legs are fully mobile
- swallowing, breathing, urinating
- fat being deposited beneath wrinkled skin
- body covered by lanugo

Week 19   Your baby may be able to hear your voice and feel your touch, as the brain designates specific areas for each of the senses—smell, vision, touch, taste, and hearing. If you feel like it, interact with him by speaking, singing, or reading aloud. Effleurage can be practiced now and will be helpful when labor begins. Effleurage involves lightly massaging your abdomen with your fingertips in circular, rhythmic strokes. The massage itself can help you relax by concentrating on the rhythm and movement. This will aid in helping your brain "forget" the pain response, which can help you feel more comfortable during labor.

Your baby is developing the ability to suck, which will be necessary for feeding once he is born. It's possible thumb sucking started even before birth.

The toes and fingers have developed distinct patterns in the skin. Even between identical twins, these fingerprints and footprints are now distinct and permanent.

His scalp is beginning to sprout hair.

Your baby is about the size of a tomato, weighing 8.5 ounces, and CRL measuring 6 inches.

Week 20   As the fetus develops the ability to swallow and digest, meconium begins to accumulate in the intestines. The taste buds can now communicate taste signals to her brain, and she is ingesting food molecules that have made their way from your blood into your amniotic fluid. Although it's unclear whether babies can taste these molecules, some research suggests the foods you eat while pregnant may affect the foods your baby later prefers.

The development of human egg cells begins in female fetuses. The testes of male fetuses wait in the abdomen until the third trimester, when they will begin to descend to the groin.

The fingernails grow toward the ends of the fingers.

Your baby is about the size of a banana, weighing 13.08 ounces, and CRL measuring 6.37 inches.

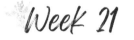 **Week 21** The flutters and stabs the fetus used to make against the walls of your womb have turned into full-on kicks and jabs. As you become more familiar with his behavior, you may begin to notice patterns.

The previously mentioned fine, downy hair, known as lanugo, has now completely covered his body.

The majority of the blood cells up until this point have been produced by the fetal liver. The bone marrow begins to assist with this task and takes over as the main source of red blood cells by Week 24.

Eyebrows are visible.

Your baby is swallowing and urinating more.

Fingerprints are now permanent.

Your baby is about the size of a carrot, weighing 14.1 ounces., and CRL measuring 6.81 inches.

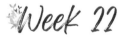 **Week 22** The fetus now looks like a miniature newborn. Lips and brows are more distinct, as are other fine features.

A stethoscope can now pick up the heartbeat.

Her eyes are open and have a pupillary response to light, but they still lack the pigment that will give them color. Tear ducts are starting to develop.

The sounds coming from inside your body, such as your breathing, heartbeat, and digestion, can be heard by the fetus and can cause her to respond. As her hearing improves, these sounds will become louder. Using a sound machine that produces whooshing and thumping noises that are familiar to your newborn and may help her sleep better.

Your baby begins to move independently. She can now touch one hand with the other and reach for the umbilical cord.

In boys, the testicles are starting to descend into the scrotum.

Your baby is about the size of a spaghetti squash, weighing 0.87 pounds, and CRL measuring 7.25 inches.

~

Month 6

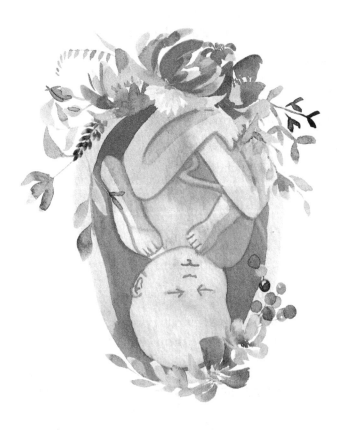

Your baby's skin is reddish in color, wrinkled, and has visible veins. At this stage, his brain is growing quickly.

Your baby moves or quickens its heartbeat in response to sounds. You may notice jerking motions if he hiccups.

Although they are formed, the fetal lungs are not yet fully developed. A premature baby may survive with intensive medical care if born at 24 weeks, the age of viability.

Overview and highlights:

- Sounds may be heard
- Sense of touch developed
- Lungs with rudimentary function
- Scalp hair
- Eyes opening
- Visible fingerprints

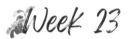 In addition to gaining more muscle and fat, the fetal lungs continue to grow and develop with growing blood vessels. You may notice more movement than in prior weeks because his muscles are strengthening and he is beginning to move around more.

Your baby is capable of hearing loud noises like a dog barking as well as sounds coming from outside your body, like your voice or that of your partner. According to research, babies begin to recognize and clearly prefer their mother's voice over others while still inside the womb.

Wave-like motions are present in his digestive tract. Since there isn't any food to move at the moment, it is merely practice for the digestive system, similar to swallowing.

Your baby is about the size of a large mango, weighing 1 pound, and CRL measuring 7.62 inches.

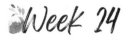 This week is regarded as the "age of viability" for preterm infants. A high-level NICU setting and immediate life-saving interventions are now necessary for the survival of these babies. They could still run into both short-term and long-term issues even with the best care. It is difficult to determine a specific age at which a baby born very, very early can absolutely survive because fetal viability depends on a wide range of variables.

The fetal lungs are developing and increasing the number of respiratory sacs (alveoli) at the tips of the tiniest branches, increasing the surface area available for the exchange of oxygen and carbon dioxide. Surfactant begins to be produced in the fetal lungs at about 24 to 28 weeks of pregnancy. The tiny alveoli collapse with every breath if there is insufficient surfactant at birth. It becomes more difficult to breathe as damaged cells accumulate in the airways as the alveoli deflate. In an effort to re-inflate the collapsed airways, your baby works harder and harder to breathe. By Week 35, most babies have enough surfactant to survive outside of the womb without ventilator support.

Your baby is gaining weight proportionately and will soon begin to plump up. Her skin is still delicate and transparent.

Just a few weeks ago, the face began to sprout tiny eyebrows. The fetus can now practice raising those eyebrows by using her facial muscles.

The brain is connected to limbs and organs by a network of nerves that is expanding.

The internal structures of her ears have grown to an adult size and shape.

Your baby is about the size of an eggplant, weighing 1.29 pounds, and CRL measuring 8 inches.

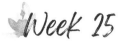 Your baby's nervous system is developing quickly and aids in his ability to move, think, and feel.

Even though the bones are continuing to harden, they are still not fully formed. Only about 80% of the skeletal system is complete.

The fetus appears more like a newborn as the baby fat begins to accumulate and smooth out the wrinkled skin.

The color and texture of his hair are starting to emerge.

The majority of your baby's time is spent sleeping, with cycles of rapid eye movement (REM) sleep and non-REM sleep occurring every 20 to 40 minutes.

Your baby is about the size of an ear of corn, weighing 1.70 pounds, and CRL measuring 8.27 inches.

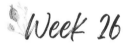 Your second trimester comes to an end this week.

Amniotic fluid is being inhaled and exhaled by the fetus in greater amounts, which aids in lung development. These breathing exercises are helpful preparation for her first breath of air at birth.

Your baby can hear a wider variety of sounds and will react by altering her breathing, movement, and heartbeat.

If you're having a boy, his testicles have begun to descend into his scrotum, a short trip that will take about two to three months.

Your baby is about the size of a bunch of scallions, weighing 1.9 pounds, and CRL measuring 8.5 inches.

MATERNAL BODY CHANGES DURING THE SECOND
TRIMESTER

As their hormones balance out, many women who battled nausea earlier in their pregnancy start feeling happier, sleeping better, and enjoying a surge of energy (Family Doctor Editorial Staff, n.d.). The second trimester is often described as the ideal time for completing tasks, such as designing and preparing the baby's nursery. Be prepared to start showing at some point in this trimester. It may be a good time to start shopping for maternity clothes, as some clothing may begin to feel a little tight around the waist. Additional bodily changes include:

Skin Changes: You may find stretch marks forming in areas such as your belly and breasts. No treatment is available to prevent this, though it is best to stick to your recommended weight gain for each trimester. In addition to stretch marks, you may find your skin feels drier and itches. You can use moisturizers to soothe itching. You may burn more easily in the sun, so wear good sunscreen when you are out and about. A linea nigra (the dark line down your belly) and melasma (dark facial patches) may appear. They tend to go away once you have given birth. This was discussed in Chapter 4 because these signs sometimes show up earlier.

Breast Growth: Enlarged milk glands and fat deposits can cause your breasts to grow. You may notice tiny bumps around your nipples, which contain an oily substance that keeps your nipples hydrated. Colostrum may start to leak from your nipples at this stage.

Aches and Pains: Your growing belly may place more pressure on your back. Meanwhile, loosening the ligaments that hold bones together in your hips and pelvis can result in pain. This change is essential, as it is your body's way of preparing for the process of childbirth. Your legs can cause pain, as your growing baby can put pressure on the nerves and blood vessels that lead to your legs, resulting in cramps. You may find that sleeping on your side rather than your back brings some relief.

Dental and Oral Changes: Pregnancy hormones can cause the ligaments and bones in your mouth to relax, but they will stiffen again after your pregnancy (March of Dimes, n.d.). It is wise to visit your dentist and diligently practice daily dental hygiene because pregnancy presents unique threats to your oral health.

Increased progesterone and estrogen levels in the body, new eating habits, and less frequent dental care since brushing and flossing can cause nausea in some women. All contribute to an increased risk of tooth decay, gingivitis, and periodontal disease. Periodontitis is a severe infection of the gums that results in teeth becoming loose and needing to be extracted. It is hazardous because it can cause bacteria to enter the bloodstream and be passed through the placenta to your baby. Smoking can cause low birth weight and increase the likelihood of serious gum disease, which is another excellent reason to quit smoking.

As Chapter 3 mentions, additional oral health issues can arise, including harmless lumps forming on the gums, usually between teeth. These tumors are red and sensitive and can bleed when brushing your teeth. They can be caused by plaque, so it is a good idea to visit your dentist for a professional cleaning.

Finally, frequent vomiting can erode your tooth enamel because vomit is acidic. If you have morning sickness, take the time to rinse your mouth after a bout of vomiting. Avoid mouthwashes that contain alcohol, since they can dry out your mouth. When there isn't enough saliva in your mouth, cavities can develop. Make your own natural DIY mouthwash by blending one cup of water and one teaspoon of baking soda (Royal Oak Dental, 2018). There is an array of alcohol-free mouthwashes available, which are a good choice.

Watch out for signs that your dental health is suffering. Typical symptoms include bad breath, loose teeth, new spaces between teeth, tooth pain, and gums that bleed easily. Don't worry about hurting your baby if you need dental work. Dental X-rays and local anesthetics are safe during pregnancy, as are some painkillers and antibiotics. Make sure to tell your dentist you are pregnant at the start of the visit.

Vaginal Discharge: The sticky, white, or transparent fluid that may have started in your first trimester may persist in the second trimester. This discharge is completely normal. See your doctor if the discharge develops an unpleasant odor, has a strange color, or is accompanied by soreness or itchiness. These are symptoms of a vaginal infection that should be treated.

UTIs: UTIs can be more prevalent during pregnancy. The first cause of more frequent UTIs is hormonal. During pregnancy, your urine has higher sugar, protein, and hormone concentrations. The second cause is the growth of your uterus, which presses on the bladder, causing the bladder to retain some urine when you urinate. You can get UTIs from other causes, such as bacteria from stool, sexual activity, and group B strep, which is intermittently present in the vagina.

See your doctor if you have any bladder infection or UTI symptoms, like a burning sensation when you urinate, colored or smelly urine, and/or abdominal pain. UTIs caused by group B strep can be transmitted to the fetus, so don't postpone a visit to the doctor if you have symptoms of an infection (WFMC Health, 2022).

Baby Flutters: As early as Week 16, you can start feeling flutters, which signifies your baby is moving around a lot! Between Weeks 14 and 19, babies can be particularly active because they still have lots of room to move around. Most women start feeling flutters around Week 20 or later, so don't worry if you don't feel them at this stage yet.

EMOTIONAL CHANGES DURING THE SECOND TRIMESTER

You may feel stronger and more energetic than ever. Take advantage and find all the information you need to make important decisions, write your birth plan, and attend childbirth classes. Remember to start asking for the physical and emotional support you will need now, during the next trimester, and once your baby is born.

The changes your body and mind undergo during pregnancy can affect your body image, mood, and strength. Surround yourself with uplifting people because tension and discord can leave you feeling drained, unmotivated, and pessimistic.

Educating yourself can boost your confidence and help you feel more in control of your pregnancy. According to studies, almost half of women do not know how long a full-term pregnancy lasts. One-third of women are unaware that premature newborns can suffer from significant health issues. These and other subjects may not be discussed in a typical childbirth class. When choosing a class, try one that offers more than just one or two hours a week, and supplement the information you receive in class with additional reading. Books, blogs, and official health websites are excellent places to start.

Bonding with Loved Ones

The second trimester is great for enjoying a babymoon with your partner, family, or friends. Get the OK from your health provider and choose a place that has always been on your bucket list. You can consider holding a gender reveal party at this stage. Don't forget to record the moment so you can share it with loved ones who live far away and can't make it. Although most providers schedule an ultrasound at around 18 to 21 weeks, your baby's gender may be visible by ultrasound as early as Week 14.

YOUR WEEK 16 PRENATAL VISIT

During your visit to your health provider in Week 16 of your pregnancy, you can expect the provider to check:

- your blood pressure
- your weight
- your fundal height, a measurement in centimeters from the top of the uterus to the pubic bone. After about Week 24, the fundal height usually matches the number of weeks of pregnancy, plus or minus 2 cm. This measurement is monitored to ensure your baby is growing steadily.

- the fetal heart rate using a hand-held Doppler ultrasound device
- fetal movement, by asking you to monitor fetal movements and report their frequency and regularity; the first fetal movements are typically felt between Weeks 16 and 22
- a urine sample for protein and glucose

Your midwife will monitor your blood pressure and urine at each subsequent prenatal appointment to ensure you are not at risk for preeclampsia or gestational diabetes. Urine tests are used to look for a host of information, including the presence of a UTI.

Amniocentesis

An amniocentesis involves using a long needle inserted through your abdomen to remove a little amniotic fluid from your uterus for testing or treatment; it is not a routine test. Testing is done to determine if a baby has a genetic disorder like Down syndrome, monitor fetal lung development, check for infections or other illnesses, determine paternity, or treat an overabundance of amniotic fluid in the uterus (polyhydramnios). This test is usually undertaken between Weeks 15 and 20.

YOUR WEEK 20 PRENATAL VISIT

In Week 20, you will have the same tests as in Week 16, that is:

- weight check
- blood pressure check
- fundal height measurement
- fetal heart rate check
- fetal movement
- urine dipstick to check for protein and sugar
- anatomy scan–the 20-week anatomy scan uses a Doppler to get a precise glimpse of your baby. The practitioner can check the baby is developing well and reassure you. They look in

detail at the baby's heart, brain, spinal cord, face, kidneys, abdomen, and bones [NHS, n.d.].

YOUR WEEK 24 PRENATAL VISIT

A month will have gone by since your last visit, and you can look forward to once again having the following assessments:

- weight check
- blood pressure check
- fundal height measurement
- fetal heart rate check
- fetal movement
- urine dipstick to check for protein and sugar

Your second trimester is one of incredible development for your baby. They have done some amazing things by the end of this stage, including smelling odors and developing eyebrows. You will notice changes in yourself, including the growth of your breasts and belly.

Non-stress Test

Your health provider may recommend you have a non-stress test (or NST) after Weeks 26 to 28 of pregnancy (Mayo Clinic, n.d.). This non-invasive test involves testing your baby's fetal heart rate. This is done by having you sit down and taking your blood pressure at various intervals. Additionally, a sensor is placed around your abdomen to test the fetal heart rate. You may have weekly or twice-weekly NSTs if you have a high-risk pregnancy. This test will be discussed in Chapter 7.

Your baby is almost here! One more trimester, and you will be holding your baby in your arms for the first time. The last and final chapter will cover your pregnancy from Weeks 27 to 40.

CHAPTER SUMMARY

During the second trimester, you and your baby will undergo tremendous changes, including:

- Your baby will grow from around 3.5 inches in Week 14 to 9.5 inches in Week 27.
- You will undergo many physical changes, including skin changes, breast growth, and dental changes.
- You will have prenatal visits around once a month, usually on Weeks 16, 20, and 24.
- You may be advised to have additional tests, such as an amniocentesis or a non-stress test.

In the next and final chapter, it's time to prepare for your baby's arrival and ensure you stay up-to-date with the many tests on your schedule.

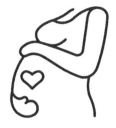

7

THE THIRD TRIMESTER

The term "watchful waiting" is often used to describe the third trimester. You are on edge as you watch and wait for the signs and symptoms of labor because you have the uneasy feeling the baby could arrive at any moment.

The development of the fetus continues to increase in size and weight during the third trimester of pregnancy. The lungs are still developing, and the fetus is starting to place itself head-down. You may experience physical and emotional difficulties throughout the third trimester. By the end of Week 37, the baby is considered full term, and delivery is just a question of time. By the third trimester, your baby's arrival will be more of a reality than ever. As you reach the last few weeks, you can start feeling more tired again, and you may be both excited and a little anxious about the day your baby arrives. You will soon have to make more frequent visits to your provider than in the second trimester and undertake new, different tests. This chapter will address how your baby will develop from Weeks 28 through 40 and examine the major physical and emotional developments you will undergo.

FETAL GROWTH AND DEVELOPMENT DURING THE THIRD TRIMESTER

Month 7

The fetal body is beginning to round out as it continues to mature and accumulate body fat reserves. The body is more proportionate because of the significant weight gain.

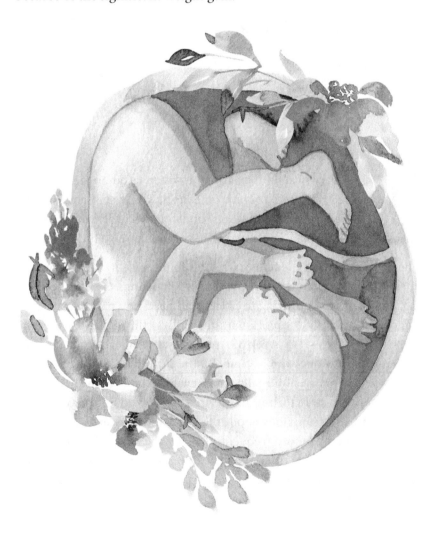

Overview and highlights:

- reddened skin covered with vernix
- responds to light, sound, and pain
- ability to taste
- hearing developed
- eyes open and close
- lanugo starts to shed

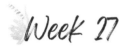 **Week 27**

Welcome to your last trimester!

By week 27, your baby looks similar to how he will appear at birth but smaller and leaner.

Your baby would have a very good chance of surviving if born now, even though his lungs have not yet fully developed. By inhaling and exhaling amniotic fluid, he keeps practicing breathing. The frequency of your baby's hiccups may increase. The hiccups are frequent at this stage because he is exhaling and inhaling increasing amounts of amniotic fluid.

Antibodies are being produced by his developing immune system.

Your baby is now growing into his own sleeping and waking patterns, so you may notice he is settling into a routine, or schedule, for when he is awake and active and when he is sleeping and being more still.

Your baby can recognize your voice as well as that of your partner as his hearing continues to develop. Because the ears are still protected by vernix, sounds may be muffled.

Your baby's eyelids open and close, and he may blink in response to light.

Your baby's skeleton continues to harden, and the bones are getting stronger. His movements are becoming more coordinated as he sucks, swallows, and blinks.

Your baby's skin is becoming less transparent.

The fetal brain is still forming and growing and is currently undergoing intense activity as neurons and synapses form intricate connections. Rapid brain growth makes his head heavier, which gradually shifts his position due to gravity. The head is most likely facing downward or in a downward diagonal at week 27. Experts assert that your baby is capable of dreaming right now, despite the lack of evidence to support this.

Your baby may react differently to different sensations as he grows. He may respond to environmental sounds and temperature changes. He may become more animated while you're out walking, hearing the sounds of the traffic or other loud noises. When drinking extremely hot or extremely cold beverages, you can anticipate him kicking more forcefully.

Your baby is about the size of a cauliflower, weighing 2 pounds, and CRL measuring 9.19 inches.

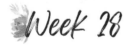 **Week 28**

The brain triples in size during the third trimester as billions of new nerve cells are formed. The largest region of the brain, the cerebrum, which controls temperature and coordinates movement, forms deep, wavy grooves that increase the surface area without adding to the volume of the skull. A protective layer of myelin begins to form around these nerves and will continue to do so for the first year of life.

Your baby's eyes are still developing, so it's possible she can detect light coming in from the outside. Her eyelashes have grown in, and she is capable of blinking. There are more rapid eye movements, linked to REM sleep. Dreams appear during this light sleep, and the eyes move quickly back and forth. Scientists have found babies in the womb may start experiencing REM around Week 23, so it is likely she begins dreaming at this point.

The senses of touch, smell, and hearing are all functional.

The intestines are growing longer and coiling inside your baby's abdomen. The length and diameter of the umbilical cord, which supplies nutrients to your baby and removes waste, are also increasing in length and diameter.

It's time for your baby to start gaining some weight for life outside the womb by adding layers of fat.

Your baby is about the size of a coconut, weighing 2.19 pounds, and CRL measuring 9.67 inches.

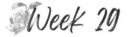 **Week 29** Your baby is putting on weight quickly, adding to his fat and muscle mass and fortifying his bones. The fetal bones absorb a lot of calcium as they harden, about 250 milligrams daily. Half of his birth weight will be gained during the last 2.5 months of pregnancy.

The fetal head occupies a significantly large portion of his body mass as it expands to accommodate his growing brain.

The skin is thickening, and the lanugo that covers his body will soon begin to shed.

Now that the eyes are open, your baby can follow moving objects. Additionally, as he grows, your baby's hearing will improve, and his ability to detect loud noises will increase.

Red blood cell production begins in the bone marrow.

If you're carrying a boy, his testicles will be moving from the abdomen into his scrotum.

Your baby will most likely be vertical and in a head-down position. If not, there is still time for him to turn, and he will be expected to do so.

Your baby is about the size of a pomelo, weighing 2.75 pounds, and CRL measuring 10.04 inches.

Week 30 Your baby is most likely head down, and she is expected to move deeper into your pelvis over the next few weeks. She is rapidly gaining weight in order to get ready for life outside the womb. Layers of fat will be added, and she will gain about half a pound weekly. Her extra fat makes her appear less wrinkled and will keep her warm after birth.

Although fetuses first hiccup at ten weeks, they are hiccupping significantly more by Week 30. The baby's diaphragm contracts as some amniotic fluid moves into her lungs during inhalation. A tiny hiccup results, which feels like rhythmic twitches in your abdomen.

A pint and a half of amniotic fluid surrounds your baby, though this amount will decrease as she grows and takes up more room in your uterus. After reaching a peak at around 34 to 36 weeks, the amount will begin to diminish. This is an indication of typical fetal growth.

The fine hair that covers her body starts to fall out, but she may have a lot of hair on her head.

Your baby's skin cells are making the pigment that gives skin its color. Babies are born a few shades lighter than their eventual skin color because melanin production doesn't begin until after birth.

Your baby can now see dim shapes but not colors, and she can distinguish light from dark. The pupils are able to constrict and expand. Your baby will turn her head in the direction of a bright light. When your baby is first born, her vision is limited to what is directly in front of her face.

Your baby is about the size of a cabbage, weighing 3 pounds, and CRL measuring 10.4 inches.

Week 31 Your baby's body is beginning to plump up as needed fat accumulates underneath his skin, smoothing out the skin and filling out his arms and legs. Get ready for a growth spurt.

All the fetal organs are now developed and functional. Organs and body systems continue to mature.

The brain has developed to the point where it can now control body heat. The neurons in the brain develop at a rapid pace during this period to ensure his brain is ready for the outside world. With less than 10 weeks left, your baby needs his brain to be in top shape to handle all the environmental stimulation. This rapid development leads to the development of the five senses: sight, smell, taste, touch, and hearing.

Your baby is swallowing large amounts of amniotic fluid and eliminating several cups of urine every day. The volume of amniotic fluid is being replaced completely several times a day.

As their survival rate dramatically increases when compared to infants born before this time, babies born during this week are regarded as being in the final week of the "very preterm" category.

At this size, the fetus can no longer flip around inside your uterus. He can still move his limbs and is still extremely active, so expect to feel lots of kicks and bumps as he moves. He can even suck his thumb, typically doing so in the fetal position.

Your baby is about the size of a zucchini, weighing 3.39 pounds, and CRL measuring 10.8 inches.

~

Month 8

The fetus keeps growing and building up reserves of body fat. Some of the wrinkles in her skin are smoothed out by these subcutaneous fat deposits.

The rhythmic breathing patterns and body temperature are under the control of the fetus.

Her bones will ossify or harden, while the four pliable bones of her skull will remain a bit softer to allow for passage through the pelvis and birth canal.

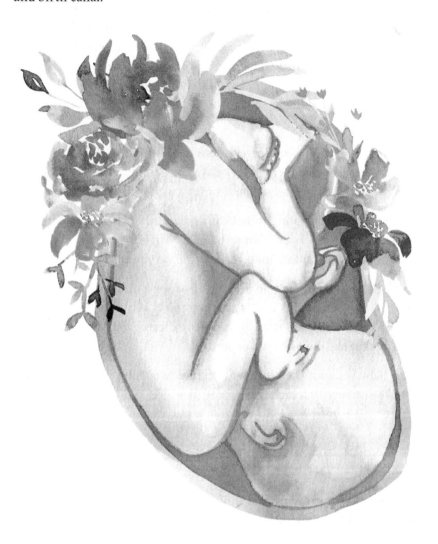

Overview and highlights:

- Skin wrinkled, little fat below the surface
- Lanugo gone from face

- Lungs developed enough to require only minimal NICU support
- Fingernails reach the ends of fingers
- Eyes open, sensitive to light

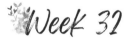 **Week 31** Your masterpiece is undergoing the finishing touches. He clearly has eyelashes, eyebrows, and scalp hair with visible color and texture. Your baby's lanugo hair, which has protected him since the beginning of the second trimester, is shedding, though some may stay on his shoulders and back when he is born. Fingernails and toenails are grown in. His skin is less transparent because of the fat deposits beneath it.

The bones, though molded into the right shape, are soft and malleable. They still need to harden.

Your baby shows signs of entering different stages of sleep and waking, and he can engage in active sleep. Slight movements can be seen while in REM, also known as "active sleep." His breathing may speed up, his eyes may move around (while closed), and his limbs and fingers may twitch or jerk.

The fetus can display the Moro startle reflex while still in the womb, though this reflex can start weeks earlier. This reflex is a hardwired response to something unexpected, like a loud sound or the sensation that they are falling. When the trigger occurs, the baby flings his arms up and out and opens his hands. Then, he draws his arms back to his body and relaxes.

Most babies born at this age are healthy and do not require any special intensive medical care. However, some babies may need to be monitored closely or admitted to the neonatal intensive care unit for further observation and treatment.

Your baby is about the size of a head of lettuce, weighing 3.83 pounds, and CRL measuring 11.2 inches.

. . .

Week 33   Your baby is still growing and gaining weight as you get closer to your due date. During this time, she gains half a pound weekly. Your baby's body will continue to fill out with fat for warmth and protection. Her skin is becoming less transparent and red, and she is rapidly losing that wrinkled, alien appearance. It's getting softer and smoother as she bulks up.

The bones in your baby's skull aren't fused yet. That allows them to shift and overlap as her head squeezes through the birth canal. Those bones won't fully fuse until adulthood, so they can grow as the brain and other tissues expand during infancy and childhood.

In these last few weeks before birth, the billions of developed neurons in your baby's brain are helping her to learn about the in-utero environment—your baby can hear, feel, and even see a little. Her eyes can detect light, and the pupils can constrict and dilate in response to it.

Your baby already has her own immune system. Antibodies are passing from you to her as he continues to develop.

Like a newborn, your baby sleeps much of the time and even has rapid eye movement (REM) sleep, the sleep stage during which our most vivid dreams happen.

Your baby's lungs are almost completely mature.

Your baby is about the size of a pineapple, weighing 4.03 pounds, and CRL measuring 11.48 inches.

Week 34   Your baby's development is almost complete. Most of the central nervous system and fetal organs are now fully formed and mature, except the lungs where primitive alveoli are formed; mature alveoli will develop later.

As the fat continues to be stored beneath the skin, your baby is beginning to look a little plumper and you can start to make out some of his first distinctive facial features. The facial features are now clearly recognized.

Your baby's brain is developing quickly, and as a result, he can learn and retain more information.

He can open his eyes and see light.

The vernix covering your baby's skin thickens as birth approaches.

During this week, when the amount of amniotic fluid surrounding your baby is at its peak, he is still swallowing it and breathing it in. This activity aids in the development of his lungs, bones, muscles, and digestive system. Temperature regulation, infection prevention, lubrication, and umbilical cord support are just a few of the crucial jobs performed by the amniotic fluid.

Babies born during this week are considered "late preterm." They may look like full-term babies, but they are still maturing.

Your baby is about the size of a cantaloupe, weighing 4.85 pounds, and CRL measuring 11.75 inches.

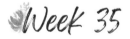 **Week 35** Your baby is now feeling very cozy inside your uterus. Due to limited space, somersaults are being replaced by forceful kicks and jabs.

She won't grow much more in length, but she'll spend the next few weeks putting on weight, gaining about half a pound per week. The majority of her weight gain now comes from fatty tissue, which will aid in her ability to control her body temperature once she is born. The significant amount of fat that is growing on her shoulders will protect this area during delivery.

However, just because your baby is almost ready for the world does not mean she has stopped developing. To give your baby's organs the best chance of maturing completely, these final few weeks are crucial.

Your baby's lungs and brain are still developing. Her brain weighs only two-thirds of what it will be at 39 to 40 weeks.

Your baby is regularly practicing her sucking reflex.

Now that your baby's kidneys are fully developed, they produce sterile urine that mixes with the rest of the amniotic fluid. For boys, the testicles should be descending by this point.

Your baby is currently floating in only a quart of amniotic fluid. Amniotic fluid production will continue to diminish until delivery.

The lanugo is almost completely gone, but the vernix coating on her skin is getting thicker.

As your baby descends low into your pelvis and relieves pressure on your lungs, any shortness of breath you were experiencing should subside (lightening).

Since they are almost ready for birth, babies born this week are categorized as "late preterm." After birth, they may require some assistance with oxygen, but they have a 99% survival rate.

Your baby is about the size of a honeydew melon, weighing 5.1 pounds, and CRL measuring 12.23 inches.

~

Month 9

This is it. Your last month.

Your baby is still maturing and growing. His lungs are now almost fully developed.

As your baby puts on a little weight, including brown fat, his skin appears less wrinkled. Waiting for labor to start naturally is preferable because this month his brain will experience a significant growth spurt. Usually, as birth approaches, your baby will either assume a head-down position or have already done so.

The fetus has coordinated reflexes that allow it to respond to sounds, light, and touch as well as blink, close its eyes, turn its head, and grasp firmly.

Skin varies in color from white to pink to blueish-pink, regardless of race (melanin is produced only after exposure to light).

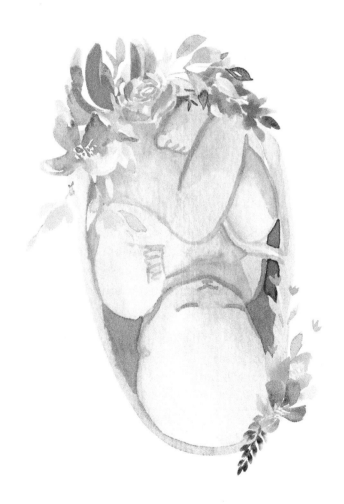

Overview and highlights:

- full growth and development are attained
- wrinkled skin has smoothed with fat deposition beneath
- lanugo has mostly disappeared
- vernix thick, disappearing
- nails project beyond fingers and toes
- left testicle has descended in scrotum

Week 36

Your baby is quickly gaining weight at a rate of roughly an ounce per day. The days of fused eyelids and lean limbs are long gone. The tiny, wrinkled fetus you first saw on ultrasounds is quickly developing into a chubby baby with chipmunk cheeks. She can open her eyes, suck her thumb, breathe, and recognize voices!

There are nails on your baby's toes now.

The vernix that shielded your baby's skin during her long amniotic soak is being shed, along with the majority of her downy lanugo coat. She swallows both of these along with other secretions, producing the meconium that will make up the contents of her first greenish-black, sticky bowel movements.

Your baby's skull bones can move and overlap each other. This ability to mold the head is necessary to enable the head to pass through the pelvis and the birth canal. Most babies are born with pointy heads to varying degrees, but don't be alarmed. Your baby's head will resume its normal shape after a few hours or days.

Your baby is about the size of a papaya, weighing 5.77 pounds, and CRL measuring 12.7 inches.

Week 37

Your due date may be three weeks away, but your baby is now considered full term. You can go into labor any day now and have a healthy baby without prematurity concerns.

Your baby's circulatory system is complete, and his bones and muscles are ready for the journey ahead.

Your baby's liver, lungs, eyes, and ears need two more weeks to fully function. His brain will grow by one-third between now and birth.

Many newborns have a full head of hair at birth, with hair ranging in length from "peach fuzz" to 2 inches. Usually, it eventually falls out and grows back in a different color.

Your baby is about the size of a head of romaine lettuce, weighing 6.3 pounds, and CRL measuring 12.98 inches.

Week 38

Your weight gain may have slowed down or stopped. This is not the case with your baby. More fat accumulates, especially around her knees, elbows, and shoulders.

Fingernails and toenails are now fully formed. By now, the lanugo will be gone, or nearly gone.

Your baby is still swallowing amniotic fluid, which is causing meconium to accumulate in the intestines.

Are you curious about the color of your baby's eyes? Because their irises—the colored portion of the eye—don't have full pigmentation yet, you may not be able to tell right away. By the time she is nine months old, her steel-gray or dark blue eyes may still be gray or blue, or they may change to green, hazel, or brown. If she has brown eyes at birth, they are likely to remain brown.

One of the reasons it's important to deliver at full term or as close to full term as possible is that your baby's brain, lungs, and liver continue to develop in the final weeks of pregnancy.

Your baby is about the size of a bunch of Swiss chard, weighing 6.46 pounds, and CRL measuring 13.35 inches.

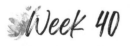 Your baby is nearing his expected birth weight during this final stage of your pregnancy. Even though his growth may have peaked, he is still undergoing some internal changes to prepare him for life outside of himself. All of your baby's organs, including the lungs, are fully formed and prepared to breathe and cry.

Since there isn't much space to move around, you may observe less fetal activity now.

Your body has been supplying your baby with antibodies through the placenta that will support his immune system during the first 6 to 12 months of life.

New skin cells are forming underneath as the surface skin cells slough off.

Umbilical cords are generally half an inch thick and about 22 inches long, which may become tangled around a baby's neck (nuchal cord). This happens quite often, but it can be easily handled at birth without any problems.

Your baby is about the size of a small watermelon, weighing 7 pounds, and CRL measuring 13.68 inches.

Week 40 Your baby is finally here after months of waiting and planning! Or perhaps not, as the majority of women don't give birth exactly on their predicted due dates. For many first-time mothers, the wait for their child to arrive can last up to two weeks after the due date.

Babies are rarely born on their actual due date. The due date is just a time that has been determined using population averages, such as the 28-day menstrual cycle. The majority of women deliver their babies within the two weeks prior to or following their due date. If you're past your due date, you may not be as late as you believe, particularly if you based your calculation solely on the day of your most recent period. Women who have longer cycles will ovulate later than expected, extending the due date accordingly.

Your body has done all it can to nourish him and now awaits the tell-tale signs that he's making an entrance. Your baby is ready to meet the world at this point.

Your baby is about the size of a small pumpkin, weighing 7.5 pounds, and CRL measuring 14 inches.

MATERNAL BODY CHANGES DURING THE THIRD TRIMESTER

Your baby is growing in leaps and bounds this trimester, and you may feel tired as your belly grows, have false labor contractions, and get ready for your baby's birth. As the baby starts to take up more space in your abdominal cavity, you may find it harder to sleep comfortably, and you may find it a little harder to take deep breaths. Midwives and other health professionals often recommend starting childbirth classes at this time (Stanford Children's Health, n.d.).

Typical bodily changes include:

- feeling slightly warmer since the fetus can radiate body heat from within
- a more frequent need to urinate
- swollen face, hands, and ankles
- more frequent leg cramps
- worse backaches in earlier weeks
- continued issues such as stretch marks, colostrum leakage, dry/itchy skin, heartburn, constipation, hemorrhoids, varicose veins, white vaginal discharge, hemorrhoids, and skin pigmentation
- Braxton-Hicks contractions may begin and come at regular intervals in preparation for the birth

- lower than usual sex drive
- coarser hair on your arms, legs, and face is attributed to the stimulation of your hair follicles by hormones

EMOTIONAL CHANGES DURING THE THIRD TRIMESTER

As your delivery day approaches, it is normal to feel stressed, especially if this is your first pregnancy. You may be concerned about not noticing signs of labor or having complications during delivery. Some women feel a little frustrated, as tiredness and their growing baby bump can make it more challenging to complete daily tasks. It is essential that you have people around with whom you can share your thoughts and emotions. Attending childbirth classes is key, as this information can enable you to approach the big day confidently and securely.

YOUR WEEK 28 PRENATAL VISIT

This visit is similar to those you have had before, though you will have new tests done. Tests are the same as those you have already had and will check:

- your weight
- blood pressure
- fundal height
- fetal heart rate
- fetal movement

All of the above will take place during the examination phase of the visit. You will have lab tests, including:

- a urine dipstick to look for the presence of protein and sugar
- a blood test to check for anemia. If you are carrying more than one baby, you should have an extra blood test at 20–24 weeks [Tommy's, n.d.].

Gestational Diabetes (Or Oral Glucose) Screen

This test is done between Weeks 24 and 28 and takes approximately two hours to perform. It takes place after you fast for eight to 10 hours, so you will usually be slotted in early in the day before breakfast. First, you will have a blood test. Next, you will be given a glucose drink and asked to rest for two hours. After this waiting period, you will have another blood test to see how your body is responding to the glucose.

RhoGAM for Rh-Negative Women if the Biological Father Is Rh-Positive

During your first trimester, your blood was tested to see if you are Rh-positive or Rh-negative. As noted in Chapter 5, if you are Rh-negative and the biological father of your baby is Rh-positive, your baby could inherit their father's positive Rh factor. This could be life-threatening for your baby, as your immune system would treat your baby's Rh-positive fetal cells as "enemies" and make antibodies to destroy them.

If this is the case, you will receive RhoGAM. This injectable medication will stop your body from making antibodies that could harm your baby. RhoGAM is routinely given at various times during pregnancy, including:

- Weeks 26 to 28, when the placenta becomes thinner and—although unlikely—blood can transfer from the mom to her baby
- within 72 hours of delivery, if the baby is Rh-positive
- after invasive testing of the baby, such as amniocentesis and chorionic villus sampling

YOUR PRENATAL VISITS IN WEEKS 30, 32, AND 34

During your prenatal visits in Weeks 30, 32, and 34, you will once again be examined to check the following:

- your weight
- blood pressure
- fundal height
- fetal heart rate
- fetal movement

You will have a urine dipstick test for protein and sugar.

YOUR WEEK 36 PRENATAL VISIT

The Group B Strep Test

During your prenatal visit in Week 36, you will have all the tests undertaken in Weeks 30, 32, and 34, plus a Group B strep test. This test can be taken between Weeks 35 and 37. The test is painless and very simple to undergo. It involves using sterile cotton swabs to collect samples from the vagina and rectum. The samples are then tested for Group B strep, a type of bacteria often found in the urinary and reproductive tracts and the digestive system.

About one in four pregnant women will test positive for GBS. This can cause infections in the amniotic fluid, womb, placenta, and urinary tract. Even if you have no symptoms, you can pass this infection to your baby during labor and delivery. Premature babies can be even more vulnerable to GBS infection than full-term babies because their immune systems are not yet developed.

If you have GBS, you will receive intravenous antibiotics every four hours during labor to kill the bacteria. Ideally, you should receive at least one dose before delivery.

YOUR PRENATAL VISITS IN WEEKS 37, 38, 39, AND 40

Once again, you will be going through a familiar routine. That includes the usual examinations and a urine dipstick test for protein and sugar.

YOUR WEEK 41 PRENATAL VISIT

In Week 41, you will have all the usual examinations, including a urine dipstick test for protein and sugar and the non-stress test. This test is usually done if you are past your due date or have a high-risk pregnancy. It takes between 20 and 60 minutes and is painless and straightforward to carry out (Mayo Clinic, n.d.).

During the NST, you lie on a reclining chair, taking your blood pressure at several intervals. Your health provider places a sensor around your abdomen to test the fetal heart rate. The test can take 20 minutes if your baby is active. If the baby is asleep, the test may need to be extended for another 20 minutes.

A reactive result, in which your baby's heartbeat speeds up to a particular level above the baseline twice or more for at least 10 seconds in 20 minutes, is the best outcome before Week 32 of pregnancy. During or after Week 32, an ideal result involves your baby's heart rate accelerating to above the baseline twice or more for at least 15 seconds each within a 20-minute time frame. This test lets your provider know if further monitoring or treatment is required.

CHAPTER SUMMARY

Once again, this is a time of significant change for you and your baby. These include:

- Your baby will grow from around 10 inches in Week 28 to approximately 14.25 inches in Week 40.
- You will undergo many physical changes and start feeling tired. You may feel like you can't wait to give birth at this point.
- You will have more frequent prenatal visits and have new tests you may not have had before, including the vaginal/rectal swab test to check for Group B strep.

Help Me Spread Peace of Mind!

You're on the greatest journey of your life, and you're armed with all the information you need to give you peace of mind every step of the way.

Simply by leaving your honest opinion of this book on Amazon, you can share that peace of mind with other expectant parents. You'll guide them toward the information that gave you exactly that.

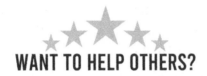

WANT TO HELP OTHERS?

Thank you so much for your support. Pregnancy is a remarkable experience—let's help other new parents relax into it and enjoy the ride.

Scan QR code for review link.

CONCLUSION

Pregnancy is a precious time in life—so much so that just a few weeks or months after giving birth, some new moms say they miss having a life growing inside their body. The sense of connection to something larger than oneself and the ability to sustain human life is profound and incomparable to any other life experience.

It can all seem unreal when you first find out you are pregnant. You can be excited but also suddenly nervous. There is so much to learn. Will 40 weeks be enough? In the beginning, you may find people eager to share their experiences with you. This is logical—after all, the birth experience is powerful, and the women in your life may want to share tips and warn you of things to avoid.

AVOIDING INFORMATION OVERLOAD

The advice can be helpful, but too many war stories contribute to fear. When talking with others, from the outset, let them know if you prefer not to hear about scary experiences, so you can feel confident as your due date approaches. When making decisions, let them be evidence-based rather than belief- or anecdote-based. Learn how to prioritize large-scale, randomized studies involving thousands of participants over small-scale or anecdotal ones.

YOU ARE NOT ALONE

You can enlist the help of a doula and have them attend childbirth classes with you. Two key elements of a positive childbirth experience are feeling confident in your choices and realizing you are not a passive subject who must accept the preferences of your healthcare providers. You can make a detailed birth plan that outlines the procedures, medications, and other components you are comfortable with and those you are not. Your choices matter.

Having a doula by your side will enable you to ask all the crucial questions that may cross your mind in the coming months, maybe regarding prenatal appointments, the birthing process, essential supplements, or physical changes like itchy skin and ankle swelling.

IMPORTANT CHOICES ABOUT BIRTH

You will be called upon to make many important decisions during this time, including whether or not to have an unmedicated delivery or one that includes pain medication. You don't have to take an all-or-nothing approach. You can use a blend of techniques that may reduce or prevent the need for pain medication. If, in the end, you do opt for an epidural or other pain management medication, you should not feel like a failure. This is just one of many decisions you will make, and it should result from carefully weighing the pros and cons.

SACRED BIRTH

For many women, pregnancy can be considered a sacred experience— a moment in time in which they see themselves as creators with a powerful ability to connect with the Earth. Sacred massage can nurture this emotion and enable you to feel more powerful. If you wish to see spirituality as an important part of your pregnancy, working alongside a midwife or doula who shares your views is important. They will help you with techniques such as breathing, which will release your fears and make you feel more grounded.

MAKING HEALTHY DECISIONS

During pregnancy, aim to take good care of yourself by eating healthy foods, staying active, and avoiding harmful substances. You should prioritize sleep and embrace activities that can help de-stress you and keep you grounded.

MAKING PRACTICAL DECISIONS

If you work outside your home or for someone else, start planning practical aspects such as your maternity leave and consider if you would like to take a more extended break to care for your baby. Think about the arrangement that will work best for your family, be it a combination of family care and babysitting or professional childcare for your baby.

BUILDING YOUR NETWORK

This is an ideal time to strengthen your network of family and friends. In the past, pregnancy, birth, and the postpartum period were considered communal affairs. The women did not feel isolated as their community gathered to support them and helped them rest and recover. Don't try to take on too many obligations at once. Remember that the postpartum period can be particularly tough on your emotions. Be vigilant for signs of postpartum depression and see a therapist if you feel your symptoms are sustained and/or moderate to severe.

TIME TO PLAN

In the end, you will have plenty of time to plan everything, from where you want to give birth to whether or not you will breast or bottle-feed your baby. An ideal time to undertake big tasks such as shopping for furniture and nursery design is in the second trimester, as you will feel energetic and ready to tackle many responsibilities.

During the first and third trimesters, you may feel slightly more tired than usual. During the last few weeks of your pregnancy, discomfort during bedtime and swelling in your ankles may make you feel like giving birth as soon as possible!

AN UNFORGETTABLE EXPERIENCE

As you reach the end of your pregnancy, remember the power of mindfulness. During this time, you will be existing while creating life. Soon, you will be bringing a new soul into the plane of existence. Still, during pregnancy, you are one with this soul, arguably closer to another human being than you ever will be. Two hearts and souls are united in flesh and blood. You have a choice between viewing your body as a physical container that nourishes a human being or seeing your pregnancy as a moment of profound transformation that connects you to a powerful life force that endures even after your body stops existing.

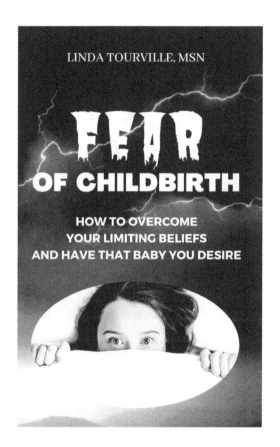

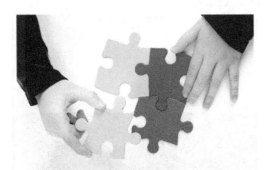

PARENTING
YOUR CHILD WITH
AUTISM

**PRACTICAL STRATEGIES TO MEET THE CHALLENGES
AND HELP YOUR FAMILY THRIVE**

LUCY TALBOTT

REFERENCES

20 best quotes about knowledge sharing. (n.d.). 30sec BLOG.

Alliance for the Improvement of Maternity Services. (n.d.). The pregnant patient's bill of rights.

Allina Health. (n.d.). First trimester: Your emotions.

American College of Nurse-Midwives. (2021, September 6). Supporting healthy and normal physiologic childbirth: a consensus statement by the American College of nurse-midwives, the Midwives Alliance of North America, and the national association of certified professional midwives. Journal of Midwifery & Women's Health 57(5), 529-532.

American College of Obstetricians and Gynecologists. (2019). Refusal of medically recommended treatment during pregnancy.

American Pregnancy (n.d.). Constipation in pregnancy.

American Pregnancy. (n.d.). Round ligament pain during pregnancy.

American Society of Anesthesiologists. (2018, May 7). Worried about the pain of labor and delivery? It's not as bad as you think!

Arguello, A. (2020, February 3). Is it normal to itch all over during pregnancy? MacArthur Minute.

Ariela. (2021, November 2). 10 causes of bleeding during pregnancy. Facty Health.

At First Sight. (n.d.). Belly binding: Cultures and beliefs.

Attachment and bonding during pregnancy. (2021, June 15). NHS inform - Scottish health information you can trust | NHS inform.

Australian Government Department of Health. (n.d.). Providing woman-centered care.

Lake, L. (2022, March 24). When and how to introduce a sippy cup. Baby Center.

Bell House Doulas. (n.d.). Midwives and doulas have similarities.

Birth Center Oak. (n.d.). Why childbirth education is important.

Birth Tools. (n.d.). What is physiologic birth?

Brian, G. (n.d.). Understanding the fear-tension-pain cycle. Birth Day Doula Co.

Budin, W. C. (2001). Birth and death: opportunities for self-transcendence. The Journal of perinatal education, 10(2), 38–42.

Cards Dental. Is dental anaesthesia safe during pregnancy? Cards Dental.

Cedars Sinai. (n.d.). Back pain during pregnancy.

Childbirth Connection. (n.d.). Birthplace basics.

Childbirth Connection. (n.d.). Making informed decisions.

Cleveland Clinic. (n.d.). Transcutaneous electrical nerve stimulation (TENS).

Cleveland Clinic. (n.d.). Medicine guidelines during pregnancy.

De Souza, R. (2016, June 11). Providing culturally safe maternal and child healthcare. Ruth De Souza.

Descisciolo, G. (2017, G). Maya prenatal massage.]

Ding, K. (2021, March 8). Breast changes during pregnancy. Baby Center.

Escobar, N. (2018, April 25). The truth behind America's soaring c-section rate. The

Bump.

Family Doctor Editorial Staff. (n.d.). Changes in your body during pregnancy: Second trimester.

Gates, M. (2021, September 13). Baby product must-haves: A list for first-time parents.

Ghandali, N. Y., Habibi, A., & Chergahian, B. (2021, July 2). The effectiveness of a Pilates exercise program during pregnancy on childbirth outcomes: a randomised controlled clinical trial. BMC Pregnancy and Childbirth, 21(480).

Glover, A. (n.d.). 5 reasons why you need a postpartum support network. The American College of Obstetricians and Gynecologists.

Graduate Nursing. (n.d.). What is a midwife?

Hainutdzinava, N., Weatherstone, K., & Worobey, J. (2017, June 12). Food cravings and aversions during pregnancy: a current snapshot. Journal of Pediatrics and Mother Care, 2(1). 110.

Harbour City Doulas. (2020, April 28). The fear, tension, pain cycle.

Hawkes, M. (n.d.). Threshold of pain. Hawkes Physiotherapy.

Healthline, (n.d.). How painful is childbirth, really?

Honor Health. (n.d.). Dealing with hemorrhoids during pregnancy.

Horbar, L. (2020, February 7). How often should you floss? 209 NYC Dental.

Johnson Memorial Health. (2015, January 15). 5 Different types of childbirth and delivery methods you should know.

Johnson, T. C. (2020, August 30). Your pregnancy week by week: Weeks 35-40. Grow by WebMD.

Jones, S. (n.d.). Who decides whether you have a caesarean section? Made for Mums.

Kids Health. (n.d.). 10 things might surprise you about being pregnant.

Kids Health. Staying healthy during pregnancy.

Klick Wire Editor. (2015, May 6). 92% of consumers like having more control over health decisions. Klick Health.

Laker, R. C., Altintas, A., Lillard, S., Zhang, M., Connelly, J. J., Sabik, O. L., Onengut, S., Rich, S. S., Farber, C. T., Barrès, R., & Yan, Z. Exercise during pregnancy mitigates negative effects of parental obesity on metabolic function in adult mouse offspring. Journal of Applied Physiology, 130(3), 605.

Legal Match. (n.d.). Pregnant patient bill of rights.

Liou, S., Wang, P., Cheng, C. (2016, August). Effects of prenatal maternal mental distress on birth outcomes. Women and Birth, 29(4), 376-380.

MacDorman, M., & Declerq, E. (2018, December 10). Trends and state variations in out-of-hospital births in the United States, 2004-2017. Birth, 46(2), 279-288.

March of Dimes. (2019). Caring for pets when you're pregnant.

March of Dimes. (2019). Dental health during pregnancy.

March of Dimes. (n.d.). Shortness of breath.

Marpie, K. (2020, April 30). The stages of labor and delivery. Baby Center.

Marvizon, J. C. (n.d.). The difference between pain and suffering. Speaking of research.

Matrix Anesthesia. (n.d.). What is the difference between an epidural and spinal block?

Mayo Clinic Staff (n.d.). Frequent Urination. Mayo Clinic.Mayo Clinic Staff. (n.d.). Prenatal care: 1st trimester visits.

Mayo Clinic. (n.d.). Nonstress test.

McCulloch, S. (2021, February 17). Meconium in amniotic fluid – Is it dangerous? Belly

Belly.

Medical News Today. (n.d.). What to know about sex during pregnancy.

MedicineNet. (2021, September 1). What are the advantages and disadvantages of a hospital birth?

Motherhood Community. (2021, January 5). A spiritual & conscious perspective on pregnancy & motherhood.

My Health Alberta. (n.d.). Childbirth: Opioid pain medicines.

National Institutes of Health. (2019, October 30). NIH-funded study suggests acetaminophen exposure in pregnancy linked to higher risk of ADHD, autism.

NCT. (n.d.). How to do perineal massage: A step-by-step guide.

Nierenberg, C., & Wild, S. (2021, May 20). Vaginal birth vs c-section: Pros and cons. Live Science.

Newham, J. J., Wittkowski, A., Hurley, J., Aplin, J. D., & Westwood, M. (2014, April 30). Effects of antenatal yoga on maternal anxiety and depression: a randomized controlled trial. *Depression & Anxiety, 31(8)*, 631-640.

NHS England. (n.d.). Involving people in their own health and care: Statutory guidance for clinical commissioning groups and NHS England.

NHS. (n.d.). 20-week screening scan.

NHS. (n.d.). Breastfeeding: positioning and attachment.

NHS. (n.d.). How to make a birth plan.

NHS. (n.d.). The stages of labour and birth.

NHS. (n.d.). Thrush.

NLBS Admin Team. (2020, April 14). *The benefits of postpartum belly binding*. New Life Birth Services.

NSW Health Pathology. (n.d.). Glucose tolerance test.

Olsson, R. (2021, August 28). When should I worry about cramping during my pregnancy? Banner Health.

Pacheco, D. (2021, March 11). Pregnancy and sleep. Sleep Foundation.

Pacheco, D. (2022, March 11). How pregnancy affects dreams. Sleep Foundation.

Pelly, J. (2022, March 10). Best online hypnobirthing classes. Verywell Family.

Penn Medicine. (2018, June 15). Varicose veins during pregnancy.

Perales, M., Artal, R., & Lucia, A. (2017, March 21). Exercise during pregnancy. JAMA, 317(11), 1113-1114.

Perry, C. (2021, August 9). Fetal hiccups: Why do babies get hiccups in the womb? The Bump.

Peterson, G. (1981). *Birthing normally: A personal growth approach to childbirth*. Shadow & Light Publications.

Pevzner, H. (2021, June 14). Your pregnancy week by week. Verywell Family.

Pregnancy, Birth and Baby. (n.d.). Braxton Hicks contractions.

Rodgers, L. (2021, October 27). What to know about the Moro reflex. What to Expect.

Royal Oak Dental. (2018, August 23). Morning sickness and your dental health.

SB Counselor. (n.d.). Understanding the difference between pain and suffering.

Schiedel, B. (2018, May 9). 17 mind-blowing ways your body changes after giving birth. Today's Parent.

Science Daily. (2008, June 3). Stretching exercises may reduce risk of pre-eclampsia during pregnancy.

Science Daily. (2011, August 28). Labor of love: Physically active moms-to-be give babies a head start on heart health.

Science Daily. (2015, November 4). Resistance exercise during pregnancy has perceived positive effects.

Seefat-van Teefelen, A., Nieuwenhuijze, M., & Korstjens, I. (2009, September 6). Women want proactive psychosocial support from midwives during transition to motherhood: a qualitative study. Midwifery, 27(1), 122-127.

Sheehy, M. (2020, January 29). How to avoid a c-section. Parents.

Shinn, L. (n.d.). 10 Comfortable Pregnancy Sex Positions for Every Trimester, Illustrated. Healthline.

Sick Kids Staff. (n.d.). Things to avoid during pregnancy: Teratogens. About Kids Health.

Spots. (2022, February 2). Pet ownership statistics.

Stanford Children's Health. (n.d.). The third trimester.Suni, E. (2021, June 24). How to determine poor sleep quality. Sleep Foundation.

Taylor, M. (2021, May 17). What is centering pregnancy? What to Expect.

The American College of Obstetricians and Gynecologists. (n.d.). The RH factor: How it can affect your pregnancy.

The American College of Obstetricians and Gynecologists. (n.d.). Travel during pregnancy.

The Spring. (2022, February 27). The importance of touch and nurturing newborns.

Thurston, J., M., & F. (2021). 1000 Questions About Your Pregnancy (5th Ed.) (Fifth ed.). JT2Books Inc.

Tolkien, Z., Stecher, L., Mander, A. P., Pereira, D. I., & Powell, J. J. (2015, February 20). Ferrous sulfate supplementation causes significant gastrointestinal side-effects in adults: a systematic review and meta-analysis. PloS One, 10(2).

Tommy's. (n.d.). Anaemia and pregnancy._.

Tommy's. (n.d.). What is hypnobirthing?

Tricycle. (2002). Pain without suffering.

Tucker, J. (2022, February 3). Is it better to naturally tear or have an episiotomy? Baby Gaga.

University of Michigan Health. (n.d.). Postpartum. First 6 weeks after childbirth.

University of Minnesota. (n.d.). What about pain?University of Rochester. (n.d.). Headaches in early pregnancy.

Varney, H., Kriebs, J. M., & Gregor, C. L. (2004). Varney's Midwifery. Jones and Bartlett Pub.

Waugh, L. J. (2011, November 1). Beliefs associated with Mexican immigrant families' practice of la cuarentena during postpartum recovery. Journal of Obstetric, Gynecologic, & Neonatal Nursing, 40(6), 732-741.

Welch, L. G., & Miller, L. A. (2008). Emotional and educational components of pregnancy. The Local Library of Women's Medicine.

WFMC Health. (2021, September 28). Swelling during pregnancy: What to expect and how to manage.

WFMC Health. (2022, February 22.). Why are UTIs so common during pregnancy?

Women's Care Staff. (n.d.). 5 common fears about giving birth. Women's Care.

Yates, S. (2017, December 28). Sacred pregnancy. Wellmother.